The Physiology of the Joints

Churchill Livingstone

Medical Division of Longman Group UK Limited

Distributed in the United States of America by
Churchill Livingstone Inc., 1560 Broadway, New York, N.Y. 10036 and
by associated companies, branches and representatives throughout
the world.

First Published 1974
   Reprinted 1975
   Reprinted 1976
   Reprinted 1977
   Reprinted 1978
   Reprinted 1979
   Reprinted 1980
   Reprinted 1982
   Reprinted 1984
   Reprinted 1985
   Reprinted 1987
   Reprinted 1988

ISBN 0-443-01209-1
Library of Congress Catalog Card Number 72 — 451799

The original French edition is entitled *Physiologie Articulaire*
and is published by Librarie Maloine, Paris.

Produced by Longman Singapore Publishers Pte Ltd.
Printed in Singapore

The Physiology of the Joints

Annotated diagrams of the mechanics of the human joints

I. A. KAPANDJI
Ancien Chef de Clinique Chirurgicale
Assistant des Hôpitaux de Paris

Translated by
L. H. HONORÉ, B.Sc., M.B., Ch.B., F.R.C.P.(C.)

Preface by
Professor R. MERLE D'AUBIGNÉ

Second Edition

Volume 3
THE TRUNK AND
THE VERTEBRAL COLUMN

1 The Vertebral Column taken as a whole
2 The Bony Pelvis and the Sacro-Iliac Joint
3 The Lumbar Vertebral Column
4 The Thoracic Vertebral Column and Respiration
5 The Cervical Vertebral Column

With 397 original diagrams by the Author

CHURCHILL LIVINGSTONE
Edinburgh London and New York
1974

PREFACE TO THE FRENCH EDITION

To understand the diseases of the musculo-skeletal system a thorough knowledge of its physiology is essential. However, its mechanical aspects, intimately concerned with the anatomy of the skeleton, have received only scant attention. The classic work of Duchenne de Boulogne concentrates only on the functions of individual muscles without specific reference to the related joints. As a result, this part of physiology, largely neglected during medical training, was little understood by surgeons, even those practising orthopaedics.

This gap has been filled now by the dedicated work of Dr. Kapandji, the artist and teacher, who has not only imagination and a flair for mechanics but also the ability to communicate his ideas in a precise and simple fashion.

His performance, already remarkable in the two previous volumes, is even more striking in the present volume which I have the honour of prefacing, since the complex movements of the vertebral column are far more difficult to understand and explain.

I feel that he has been completely successful in attaining his goal and I envy the young surgeons who have this work at their disposal. I am confident that this volume, which goes a long way towards explaining the basic mechanics of the vertebral column, will help greatly in improving the treatment of lesions of the vertebral column.

Professor R. MERLE D'AUBIGNÉ.

To My Wife

I.A.K.

CONTENTS

THE CERVICAL VERTEBRAL COLUMN

THE VERTEBRAL COLUMN AS A WHOLE

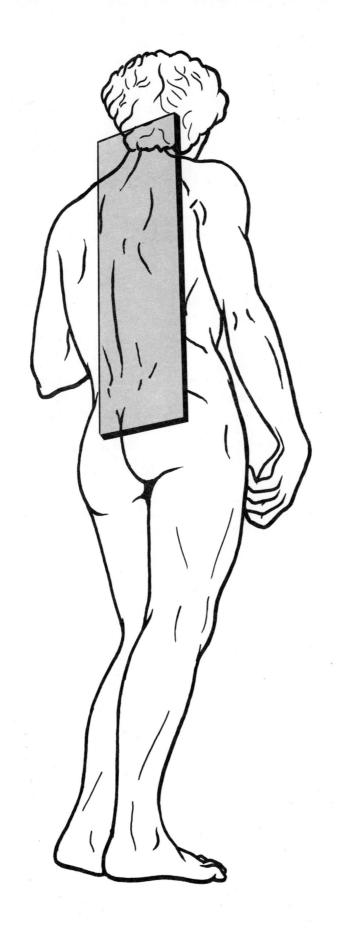

THE VERTEBRAL COLUMN: A STABILISED AXIS

The vertebral column, the axis of the body, must meet two contradictory mechanical requirements: *rigidity* and *plasticity*. This is achieved by the presence of stays built into its very structure. In fact (fig. 1), the vertebral column as a whole can be viewed as the mast of a ship. This mast, resting on the pelvis, extends to the head and, at the level of the shoulders, supports a main-yard set transversely, i.e., the scapular girdle. At all levels there are *ligaments and muscular tighteners* arranged as **stays**, i.e., linking the mast itself to its attachment site, the pelvis. A second system of stays is closely related to the scapular girdle and is diamond-shaped with its long axis vertical and its short axis horizontal. In the *position of symmetry* the forces on either side are in equilibrium and the mast lies straight and vertical.

When the weight of the body rests on one limb (fig. 2), the pelvis tilts to the opposite side and the vertical column is forced to bend: first, in the lumbar region, it becomes convex towards the resting limb, then concave in the thoracic region and convex once more. The muscular tighteners adapt automatically to restore equilibrium and this active adaptation is under control of the extrapyramidal system, which alters the tone of the postural muscles.

The plasticity of the column lies in its make-up, i.e., *multiple components superimposed on one another* and interlinked by ligaments and muscles. Its structure can therefore be altered by the muscular tighteners while it maintains its rigidity.

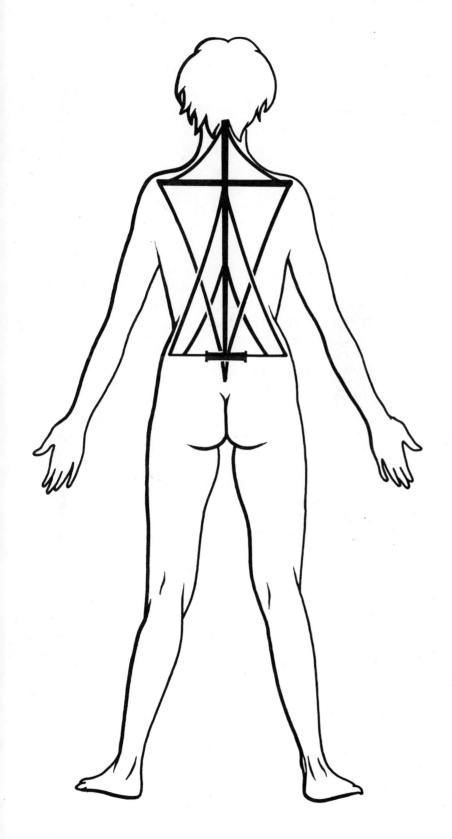

1

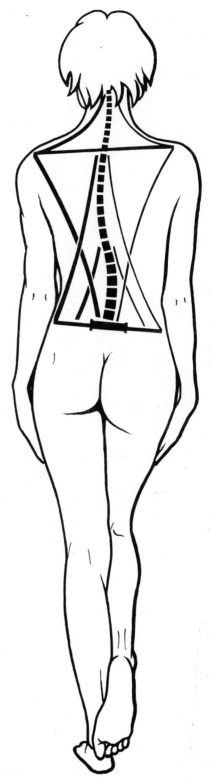

2

THE VERTEBRAL COLUMN; AXIS OF THE BODY AND PROTECTOR OF THE NEURAXIS

The spinal column in effect constitutes the **central pillar of the trunk** (fig. 3). Though in the *thorax* (inset b) it lies more posteriorly, i.e., within the posterior quarter of the thorax, in the *neck* (inset a) it lies more centrally, i.e. at the junction of the anterior two-thirds and posterior one-third of the neck. *In the lumbar region* (inset c) it lies centrally. These variations in position can be explained by local factors. In the neck the column supports the head and must lie as close as possible to its centre of gravity. In the thorax it is forced posteriorly by the internal organs, especially the heart. In the lumbar region, where it must support the whole weight of the upper trunk, it lies centrally once more and juts into the abdominal cavity.

In addition to supporting the trunk, the vertebral column **protects the neuraxis** (fig. 4): its canal, which starts at the foramen magnum and contains the medulla oblongata and the spinal cord, acts as a flexible and efficient casing. However, this protection afforded to the spinal cord is not absolute and, at certain levels and under certain circumstances, the spinal cord and its roots can be damaged by these protective structures.

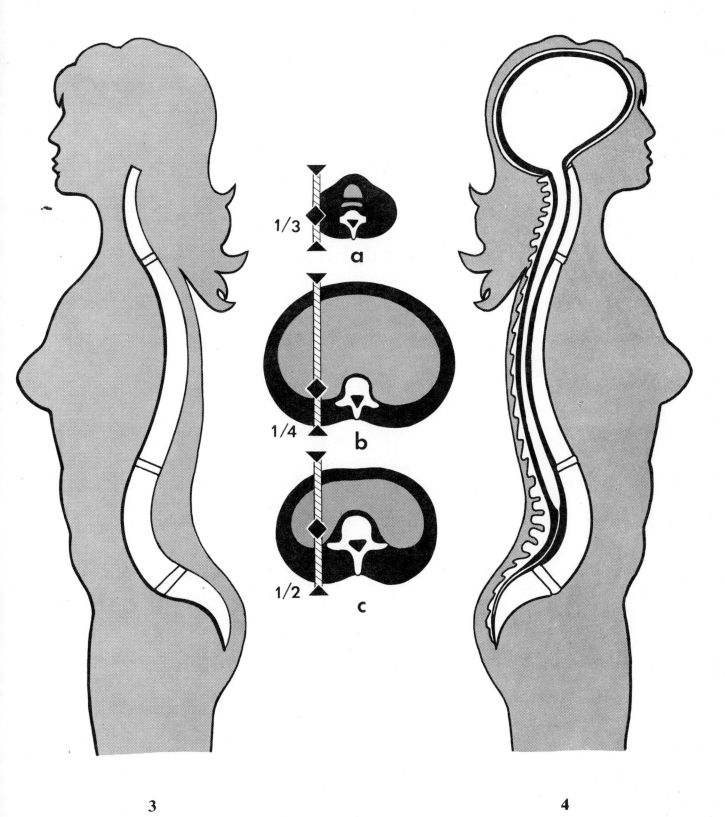

1/3

a

1/4

b

1/2

c

3

4

13

THE CURVATURES OF THE VERTEBRAL COLUMN

The vertebral column as a whole is *straight* when viewed *from the front or the back* (fig. 5). In some people, however, there may be a slight lateral curvature which remains within physiological limits.

On the other hand, *in the sagittal plane* (fig. 6) the vertebral column shows the following *four curvatures*:

1. **the sacral curvature**, which is fixed as a result of total fusion of the sacral vertebrae. It is concave posteriorly;
2. **the lumbar curvature**, concave posteriorly;
3. **the thoracic curvature**, convex posteriorly;
4. **the cervical curvature**, concave posteriorly;

When one is standing normally, the posterior part of the head, the back and the buttocks lie tangential to a vertical plane, e.g., a wall. The extent of these curvatures is indicated by the solid lines and their meaning will be discussed later.

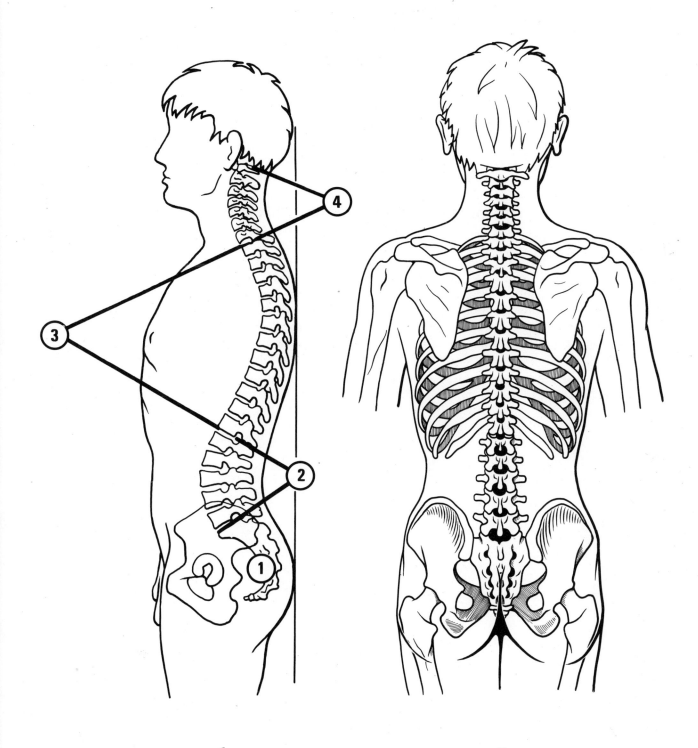

6

5

THE DEVELOPMENT OF THE CURVATURES OF THE VERTEBRAL COLUMN

During **phylogeny** (i.e., evolution), the transition from the quadruped to the biped state (fig. 7) has led first to the straightening and then to the inversion of the lumbar curvature which was initially concave anteriorly; hence the normal *lumbar lordosis* (i.e. concave posteriorly). In fact, the erection of the trunk has not been totally 'absorbed' by backward tilting of the pelvis and some contribution has come from the bending of the lumbar column. This explains the lumbar lordosis which varies according to the degree of forward or backward tilting of the pelvis.

During **ontogeny** (i.e., the development of the individual) the same changes can be observed in the lumbar region (fig. 8, according to T. Willis). On the first day of life (a) the lumbar column is concave anteriorly. At five months (b) the lumbar curve is still slightly concave anteriorly and it disappears at thirteen months (c). From three years onwards, the lumbar lordosis begins to appear (d) becoming obvious by 8 years (e) and assuming the definitive adult state at 10 years (f).

The phylogenetic changes are therefore recapitulated during ontogeny.

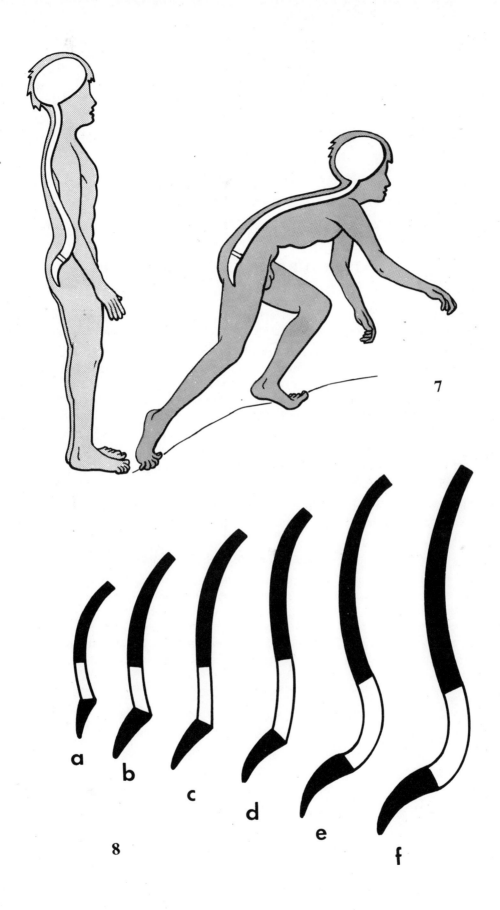

7

8

a   b   c   d   e   f

STRUCTURE OF THE TYPICAL VERTEBRA

When one analyses the structure of a **typical vertebra** (fig. 9), one finds that it is made up of two major parts, i.e., the *vertebral body* anteriorly and the *vertebral arch* posteriorly.

When the vertebra is dismantled (a) the *vertebral body* (1) is the largest part of the vertebra: it is by and large cylindrical, wider than it is tall and has a planed surface posteriorly. The *vertebral arch* (2), in the shape of a horseshoe, bears on either side (b) the *articular processes* which divide the arch into two parts: anteriorly, the *pedicles* (8 and 9) and posteriorly, the *laminae* (10 and 11). The spinous process (7) is attached to the midline posteriorly. The vertebral arch therefore is attached to the vertebral body by the pedicles. The complete vertebra (e) also bears *transverse processes* (5 and 6), which are attached to the arch near the articular processes.

This typical vertebra is found at all levels of the column with, of course, profound alterations that affect either the body or the arch but generally both simultaneously.

However, it is important to note that in the vertical plane these various constituents lie in anatomic correspondence. As a result, the entire vertebral column is made up of **three pillars** (fig. 10):

a *major pillar*, anteriorly located and made up by the stacking of vertebral bodies;

two *minor pillars*, posterior to the vertebral body and made up by the stacking of articular processes. The bodies are joined to each other by the intervertebral disc, the articular processes by arthroidal joints. Thus at the level of each vertebra there is a canal bounded by the vertebral body anteriorly and the vertebral arch posteriorly. These successive canals make up the *vertebral canal* which is constituted alternately by bony structures at the level of each vertebra and by ligaments joining the vertebral bodies and arches.

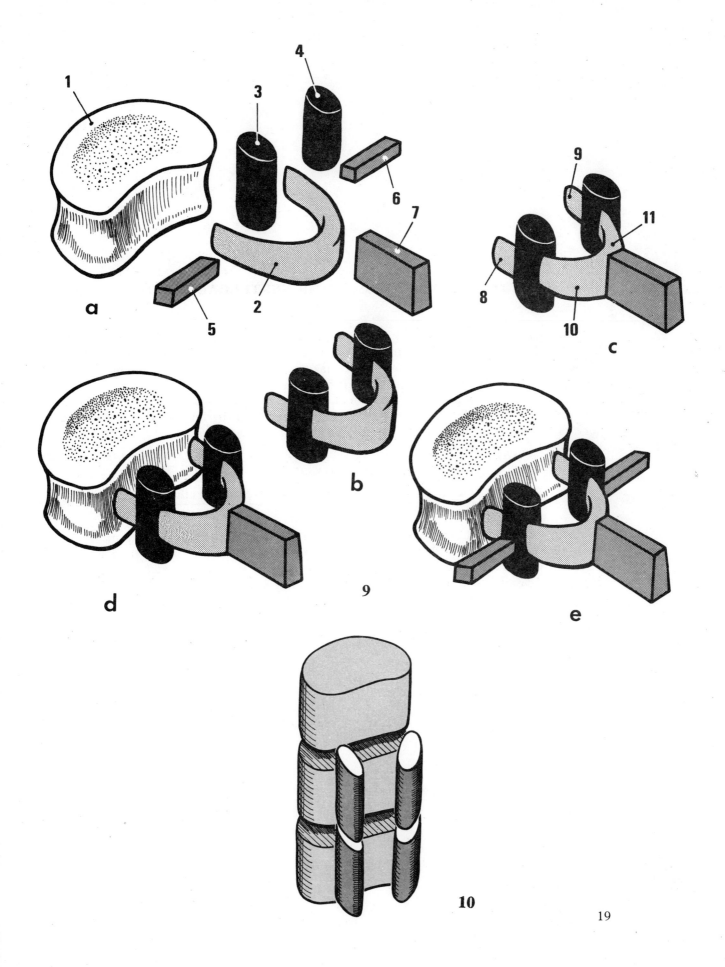

THE CURVATURES OF THE VERTEBRAL COLUMN

The curvatures of the vertebral column increase its resistance to axial compression forces. Engineers have shown (fig. 11) that the resistance of a curved column is *directly proportional to the square of the number of curvatures plus one.* If we take as reference a straight column (number of curvatures = 0), with resistance equal to 1, it follows that a column with one curvature (b) has a resistance equal to 2, a column with 2 curvatures (c) has a resistance equal to 5 and a column with 3 flexible curvatures (d)—like the vertebral column with its lumbar, thoracic and cervical curvatures—has a resistance of 10, i.e., *ten times that of a straight column.*

The significance of these curvatures can be quantitated by the **Delmas Index** (fig. 12), which can only be measured on a skeleton. It is expressed as the ratio

$$\frac{\text{actual length of the vertebral column from } S_1 \text{ to the atlas}}{\text{fully extended length of the vertebral column from } S_1 \text{ to the atlas}} \times 100$$

A column with normal curvatures (a) has an index of 95 with the limits of normality ranging from 94 to 96. A column with *exaggerated curvatures* (b) has an index smaller than 94 signifying a marked difference between the actual height of the column and its fully extended length. On the contrary, a column with *attenuated curves*, i.e., almost straight, has an index greater than 96. This anatomical classification has functional significance, as A. Delmas has shown that the column with *pronounced curvatures* is of the *dynamic* type, while the column with *attenuated curvatures* corresponds to the *static* type.

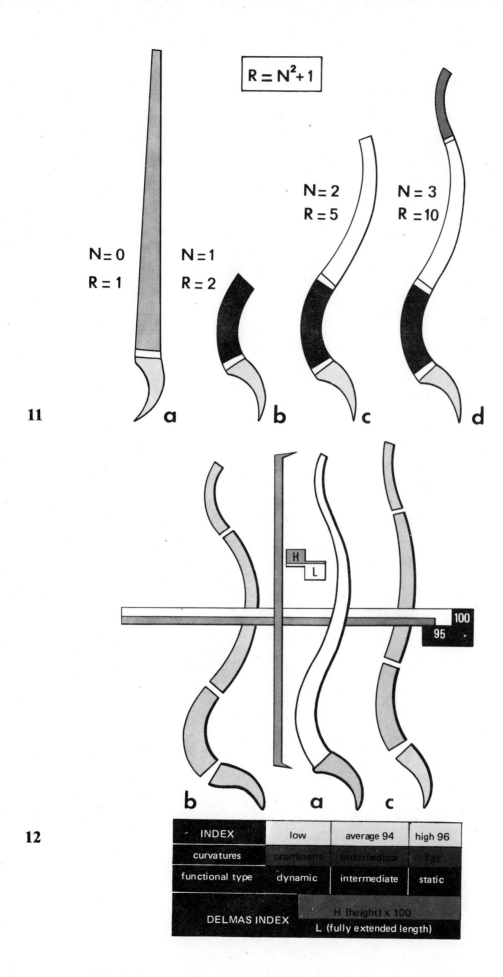

$$R = N^2 + 1$$

N= 0
R = 1

N=1
R = 2

N= 2
R = 5

N= 3
R =10

11 a   b   c   d

12

H
L

100
95

b   a   c

INDEX	low	average 94	high 96
curvatures	prominent	intermediate	flat
functional type	dynamic	intermediate	static
DELMAS INDEX	H (height) x 100		
	L (fully extended length)		

21

STRUCTURE OF THE VERTEBRAL BODY

The vertebral body is built like a short bone (fig. 14) i.e., **egg-like**, with a dense bony cortex surrounding a spongy medulla. The cortex of the superior and inferior aspects is called the *vertebral plateau*. It is thicker in the centre which contains a cartilaginous plate. The periphery is thickened (fig. 13) to form a *distinct rim*, which is derived from the epiphyseal plate and becomes fused to the body at 14–15 years of age. Abnormal ossification of this rim leads to vertebral epiphysitis (Schauermann's disease).

A section of the vertebra taken in the vertico-frontal plane (fig. 14) shows clearly: the thick cortex on either side, the cartilage-lined vertebral plateau superiorly and inferiorly, and the spongy centre of the vertebral body with bony trabeculae disposed along the *lines of force*. These lines are *vertical* linking the superior and inferior surfaces, or *horizontal* linking the lateral surfaces or *oblique* linking the inferior with the lateral surfaces.

A sagittal section (fig. 15) shows these trabeculae once more, but in addition two more sheaves of oblique fibres in *fan-like arrangement* (fig. 16 and 17). The first (fig. 16), arising from the *superior surface*, fans out at the level of the two pedicles to reach the corresponding superior articular processes and the spinous process. The second (fig. 17), arising from the *inferior surface*, fans out at the level of the two pedicles to reach the corresponding inferior articular processes and the spinous process.

The criss-crossing of these three trabecular systems constitutes zones of maximum resistance as well as a *triangular area of minimum resistance*, made up entirely of vertical trabeculae (fig. 18).

This explains the wedge-shaped compression fracture of the vertebra (fig. 19). Under an axial compression force of 600 kg the anterior part of the vertebral body is crushed, leading to a compression fracture. A similar force equivalent to 800 kg is required to crush the whole vertebra and make the posterior part give (fig. 20).

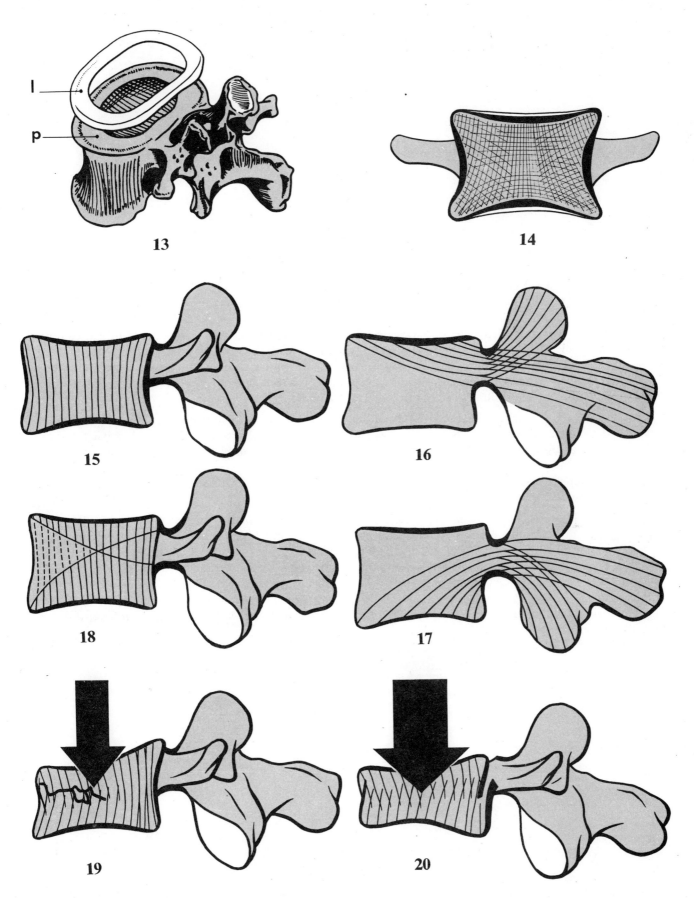

13

14

15

16

18

17

19

20

FUNCTIONAL COMPONENTS OF THE VERTEBRAL COLUMN

When viewed laterally (fig. 21, according to Brueger) the functional components of the column are easily distinguished. Anteriorly (A) lies the **anterior pillar** which is the essential supporting structure. Posteriorly lies the **posterior pillar** (B) which contains the two minor pillars (as described before), supported by the vertebral arch. While the anterior pillar (A) plays a *static role*, the posterior pillar (B) has a *dynamic role* to play.

In the vertical plane, the alternation of bony and ligamentous structures allows one to distinguish (according to Schmorl): a **passive segment** (I) formed by the vertebra itself and an **active segment** (II), bounded in the diagram by a heavy black line. It consists of the intervertebral disc, the intervertebral foramen, the articular processes, the ligamentun flavum and the interspinous ligament. The mobility of this active segment underlies the movement of the vertebral column.

There is a *functional link between the anterior and posterior pillars* (fig. 22). If one goes back to the trabecular structure of the vertebral body and arch, each vertebra can be compared to a lever system of the first order, where the articular processes (1) constitute the fulcrum. This lever system allows the absorption of axial compression forces applied to the vertebral column: *direct and passive absorption at the level of the intervertebral disc* (2); *indirect and active absorption at the level of the paravertebral muscles* (3), as a result of the lever system constituted by each vertebral arch. Therefore the absorption of compression forces is at once *passive* and *active*.

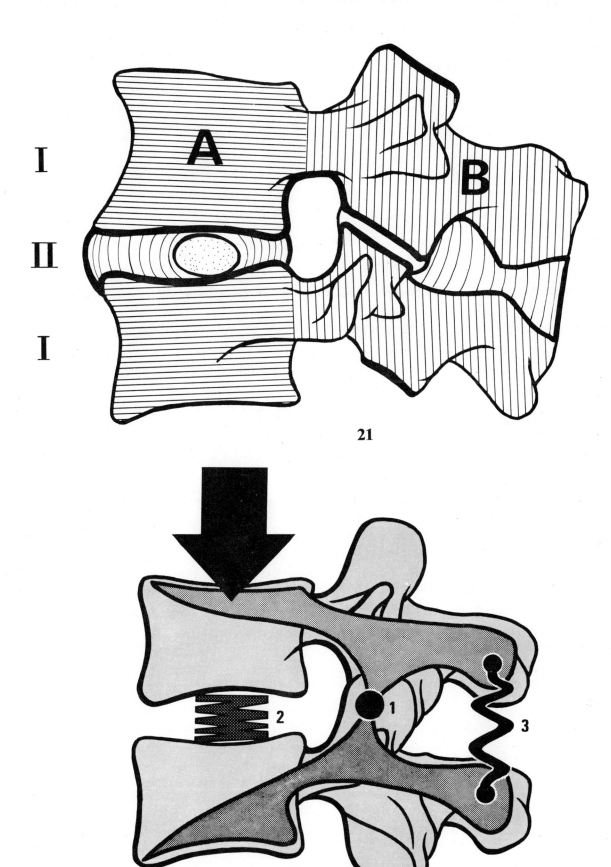

21

22

THE ELEMENTS OF LINKAGE BETWEEN VERTEBRAE

Between the sacrum and the base of the skull there are *twenty-four movable parts* linked together by fibrous ligaments.

A horizontal section (fig. 23) and a lateral view (fig. 24) show the following ligaments:

First, those attached to the **anterior pillar**.

1 *the anterior longitudinal ligament* (1), stretching from the basi-occiput to the sacrum on the anterior surfaces of the vertebrae.

2 *the posterior longitudinal ligament* (2), extending from the basi-occiput to the sacral canal on the posterior aspect of the vertebrae. These long ligaments are interlinked at each vertebral level by the intervertebral disc (D) which is made up of two parts:

peripherally, the *annulus fibrosus* formed by concentric layers of fibrous tissue (6 and 7);

centrally, the *nucleus pulposus* (8).

Attached to the vertebral arch many ligaments connect the arches of adjacent vertebrae.

The *ligamentum flavum* (3), very thick and strong, meets its contralateral counterpart in the midline and is attached superiorly to the deep surface of the lamina of the upper vertebra and inferiorly to the superior margin of the lower vertebra.

The *interspinous ligament* (4) is continuous posteriorly with the *supraspinous ligament* (5). The latter is poorly defined in the lumbar region but is quite distinct in the neck.

To the superior surface of each transverse process is attached the *intertransverse ligament* (10).

Finally, in relation to the articular processes there are two powerful *anterior and posterior ligaments* (9), which strengthen the *capsular ligaments* of the joints between these processes.

These ligaments taken as a whole maintain an extremely solid link between the vertebrae and impart a strong mechanical resistance to the vertebral column.

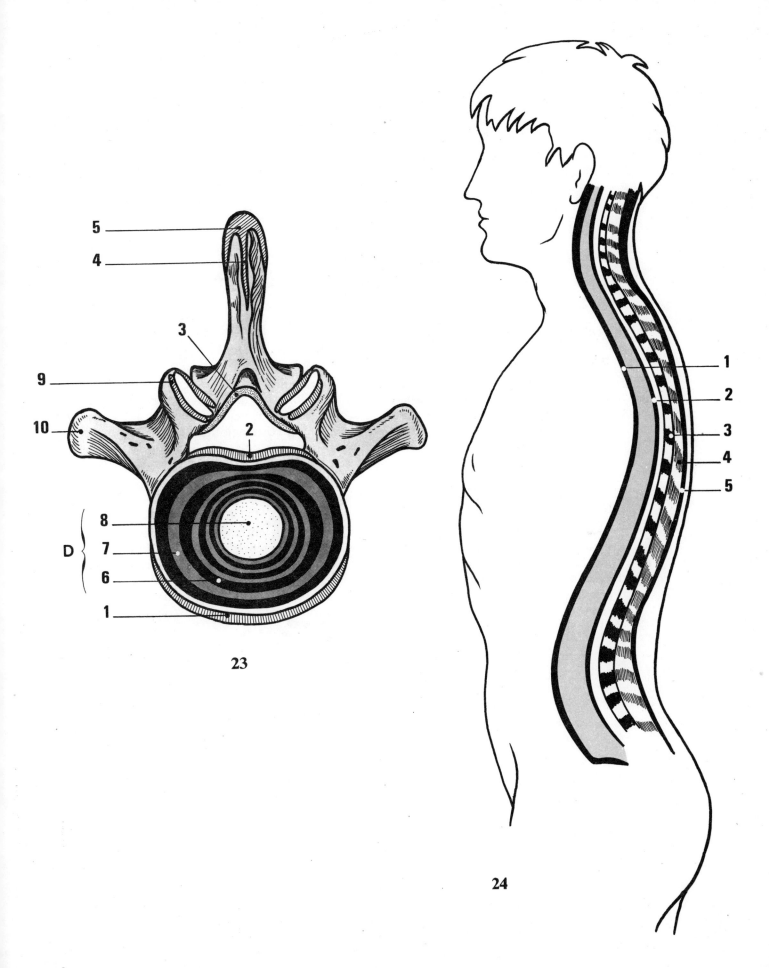

5

4

3

9

10

2

8

7

6

1

D

23

1

2

3

4

5

24

STRUCTURE OF THE INTERVERTEBRAL DISC

The joint between two vertebrae is a **symphysis**. It is formed by the two vertebral plateaus connected by the intervertebral disc. The structure of this disc is quite characteristic and consists of two parts (fig. 25):

A central part—*the nucleus pulposus* (N)— a gelatinous substance derived embryologically from the notochord. It is a transparent jelly containing 88 per cent water; it is strongly hydrophilic and chemically is made up of a mucopolysaccharide matrix containing protein-bound chondroitin sulphate, hyaluronic acid and keratan sulphate. Histologically the nucleus is comprised of collagenous fibres, cells resembling chondrocytes, connective tissue cells and very few clusters of mature cartilage cells. *No blood vessels or nerves penetrate the nucleus* which is tightly bounded peripherally by fibrous tracts.

A peripheral part—the *annulus fibrosus* (A)—made up of concentric fibres which appear to cross one another obliquely in space as shown in (a). In (b) the fibres are seen to be vertical peripherally and become more oblique towards the centre. The central fibres in contact with the nucleus are nearly horizontal running between the vertebral plateaus in ellipsoidal fashion. Thus the nucleus is enclosed within an inextensible casing formed by the vertebral plateaus and the annulus, whose woven fibres in the young prevent any prolapse of the nucleus. The latter is *held under pressure* within its casing so that, when the disc is cut, its gelatinous substance can be seen to bulge through the cut. This is also seen when the vertebral column is sectioned sagittally.

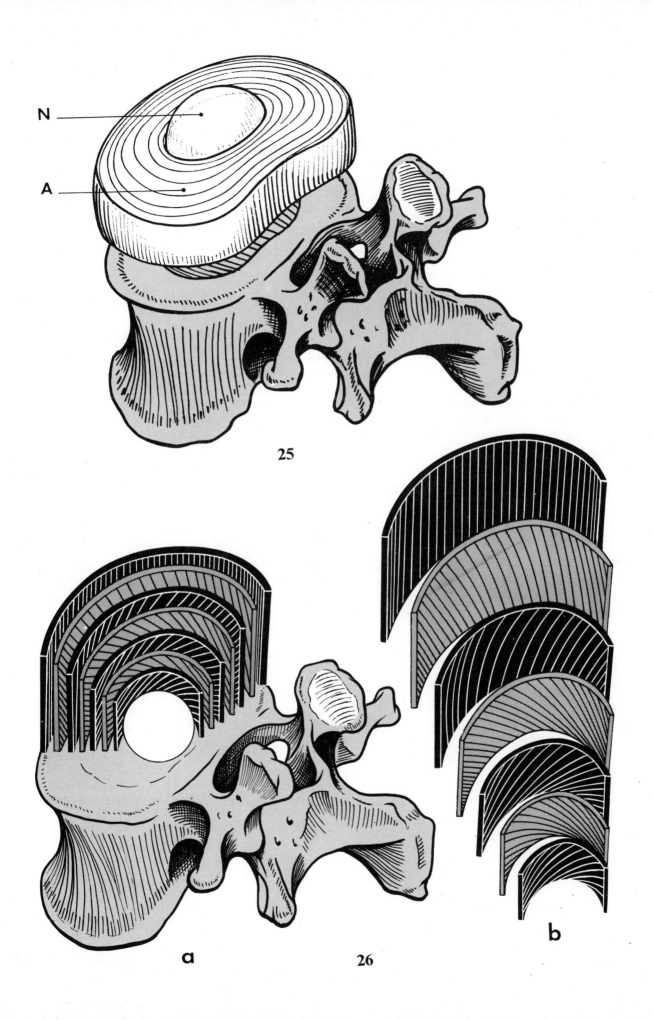

N

A

25

a   26   b

THE NUCLEUS PULPOSUS LIKENED TO A SWIVEL

Incarcerated under pressure within its casing between the two vertebral plateaus, the nucleus pulposus is roughly **spherical**. Therefore, to a first approximation, one can consider the nucleus as *a ball placed between two planes* (fig. 27). This type of joint known as a swivel joint allows three types of movement:

1 **Tilting:**
   tilting in the sagittal plane: flexion (fig. 28) or extension (fig. 29);
   tilting in the frontal plane: lateral flexion;

2 **Rotation** of one plateau relative to the other (fig. 30);

3 **Gliding and even shearing** of one plateau over the other.

Therefore, all told, this very mobile joint has **six degrees of freedom**: flexion and extension, lateral flexion, gliding in the sagittal plane, gliding in the frontal plane, rotation right and left. Each of these movements has a small range and sizeable movements are only obtained by the simultaneous participation of multiple intervertebral joints.

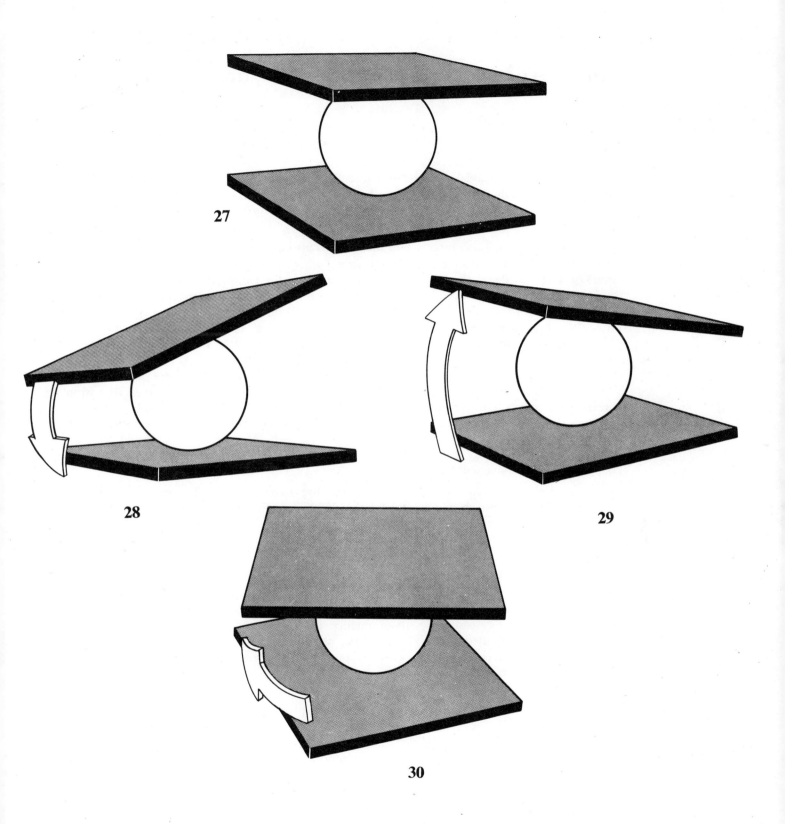

27

28

29

30

31

THE 'PRELOADED' STATE OF THE DISC AND THE SELF-STABILISATION OF THE INTERVERTEBRAL JOINT

The forces applied to the intervertebral disc are considerable, the more so as one nears the sacrum.

In terms only of axial compression forces, it has been worked out that when a vertebral plateau presses on the intervertebral disc the nucleus bears 75 per cent of the force and the annulus 25 per cent, so that for a force equal to 20 kg a 15 kg force is exerted on the nucleus and a 5 kg force on the annulus.

However, in the horizontal plane, the nucleus also *acts to transmit* some of the force to the annulus (fig. 31). For instance, *in the standing position*, at the level of L_5–S_1 the vertical compression force acting on the nucleus and transmitted to the rim of the annulus equals 28 kg/cm and 16 kg/cm². These forces are increased considerably when the subject is lifting a load. During flexion of the trunk the pressure/cm² rises to 58 kg, while the pressure/cm rises to 87 kg. *When the trunk is straightened to the vertical*, these pressures reach 107 kg/cm² and 174 kg/cm. These pressures can be higher if a weight is lifted simultaneously and they come close to the values for breaking-point.

The pressure in the centre of the nucleus is never zero, even when the disc is unloaded. This pressure is due to its water-absorbing capacity which causes the disc to swell within its inextensible casing. This is analogous to the **preloaded state**. In building technology, preloading denotes a pre-existing tension within a beam about to be stressed. If a *homogeneous* beam is exposed to a load (A), it bends inwards for a distance f_1. If a beam (B) is fitted with a taut cable passing through its inferior part, it is now **preloaded** and the distortion (f_2) caused by the same load as above will be clearly smaller than f_1.

The preloaded state of the intervertebral disc likewise gives it a greater resistance to the forces of compression and lateral flexion. With age the nucleus loses its water-absorbing capacity and the preloaded state tends to be lost; hence the lack of flexibility of the vertebral column in the aged.

When an **asymmetrical load is applied axially to a disc** (fig. 33) the upper vertebral plateau tilts towards the overloaded side, making an angle a with the horizontal. Thus the fibre AB′ will be stretched to AB but, at the same time, the internal pressure of the nucleus maximal in the direction of the arrow will bring back the fibre to position AB′ thereby righting the vertebral plateau and restoring it to its original position. This **mechanism of self-stabilisation** is linked to the preloaded state. Therefore the annulus and the nucleus constitute a functional couple whose effectiveness depends on the integrity of each component. If the internal pressure of the nucleus decreases or if the tightness of the annulus is impaired, this functional couple immediately loses its effectiveness.

The preloaded state also explains the elastic properties of the disc, as well shown by Hirsch's experiment (fig. 34). If a preloaded disc (P) is exposed to a violent force (S), the thickness of the disc exhibits dampened oscillations over a period of one second. If this force is too violent the intensity of this oscillatory reaction can destroy the fibres of the annulus. This accounts for the deterioration of intervertebral discs exposed to repeated violent stresses.

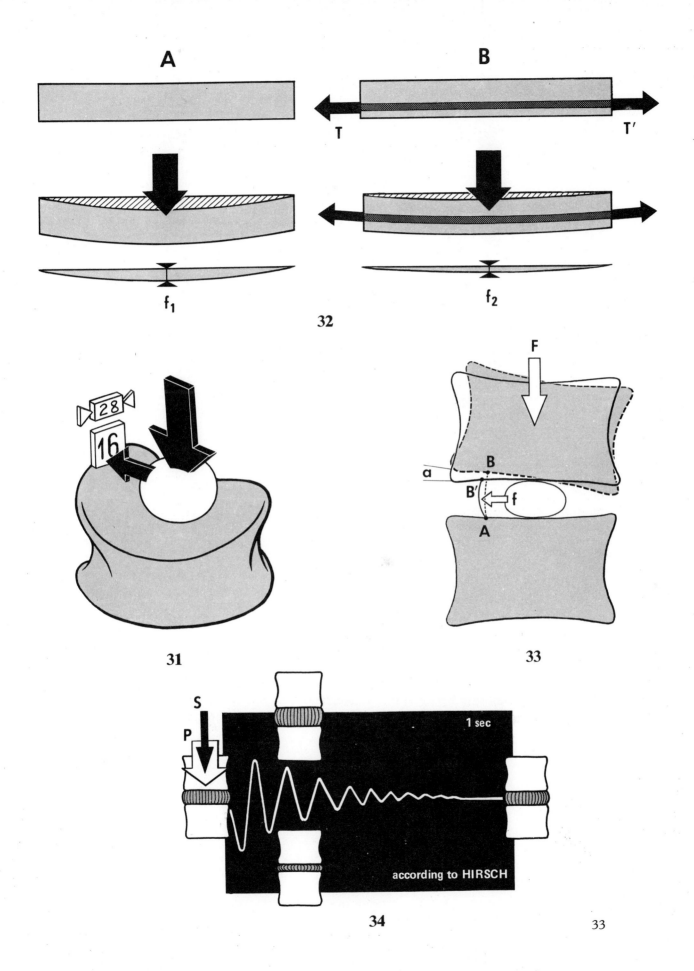

A

B

T   T'

f_1 f_2

32

31

F

a

B

B'   f

A

33

34

S

P

1 sec

according to HIRSCH

33

WATER IMBIBITION BY THE NUCLEUS

The nucleus rests on the centre of the vertebral plateau, an area lined by cartilage which is transversed by numerous microscopic pores linking the casing of the nucleus and the spongy bone underlying the vertebral plateau. When a significant axial force is applied to the column, as *during standing* (fig. 35), the water contained within the gelatinous matrix of the nucleus escapes into the vertebral body through these pores. As this static pressure is maintained throughout the day, by night the nucleus contains less water than in the morning so that the disc is *perceptibly thinner*. In a healthy individual this cumulative thinning of the discs can amount to 2 cm.

Conversely, during the night, *when one lies flat* (fig. 36), the vertebral bodies are subject, not to the axial force of gravity, but only to that generated by muscular tone, which is much reduced during sleep. At this time the water-absorbing capacity of the nucleus draws water back into the nucleus from the vertebral bodies and the disc regains its original thickness. Therefore one is taller in the morning than at night. As the preloaded state is more marked in the morning the flexibility of the vertebral column is greater at this time.

The **imbibition pressure of the nucleus** is considerable since it can reach 250 mmHg (Charnley). With age the water-absorbing ability of the disc decreases, reducing its state of preloading. This explains the loss of height and flexibility in the aged.

Hirsch has shown that when a **constant load** is applied to a disc (fig. 37) the loss of thickness is not linear but exponential (first part of the curve), suggesting a dehydration process proportional to the volume of the nucleus. When the load is removed, the disc regains its initial thickness, once more exponentially, and the restoration to normal requires a finite time. If forces are applied and removed *at too short intervals*, the disc does not have the time to regain its initial thickness. Similarly, if these forces are applied or removed over periods that are too prolonged (even if one gives enough time for restoration), the disc does not recover its initial thickness. This results in a *state analogous to ageing*.

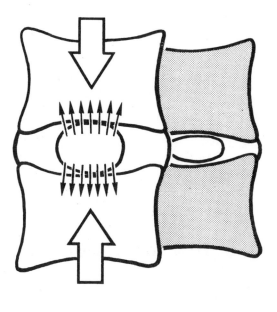

35

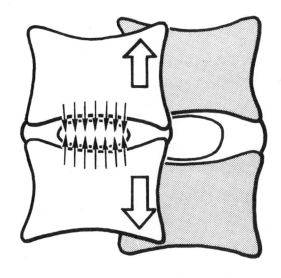

36

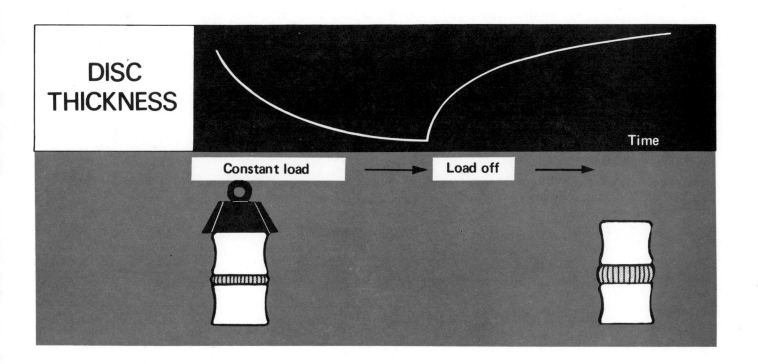

DISC THICKNESS

Time

Constant load →   Load off →

37

COMPRESSION FORCES APPLIED TO THE DISC

The compression forces applied to the disc assume greater significance the nearer the disc is to the sacrum (fig. 38), which supports the bulk of the body weight. For a man weighing 80 kg the head weighs 3 kg, the upper limbs 14 kg and the trunk 30 kg. If it is assumed that at the level of the disc L_5–S_1 the column supports only two-thirds of the trunk, the weight borne is 37 kg, which is *nearly half the body weight* (P). To this must be added the force exerted by *the tone of the paravertebral muscles* (M_1 and M_2) necessary to maintain the trunk in the erect posture at rest. If an extra load (E) or any violent overload is also added (S), the lowest discs may be subject to forces that outstrip their resistance, especially in the aged.

The loss of thickness of the disc depends on whether the disc is healthy or diseased (fig. 39). If a healthy disc at rest (A) is loaded with a weight of 100 kg it is flattened by a distance of 1.4 mm and becomes wider. If a diseased disc is similarly loaded it is flattened by a distance of 2 mm (C) and it fails to recuperate completely its initial thickness after unloading.

This progressive flattening of the diseased disc has an effect on the joints between the articular processes (fig. 40). With normal disc thickness (A) the articular cartilages of these joints are normally disposed and the interspace is straight and regular. With a flattened disc these joints are disturbed and the interspace opens out posteriorly. *This articular distortion by itself will lead to osteoarthrosis in the long run.*

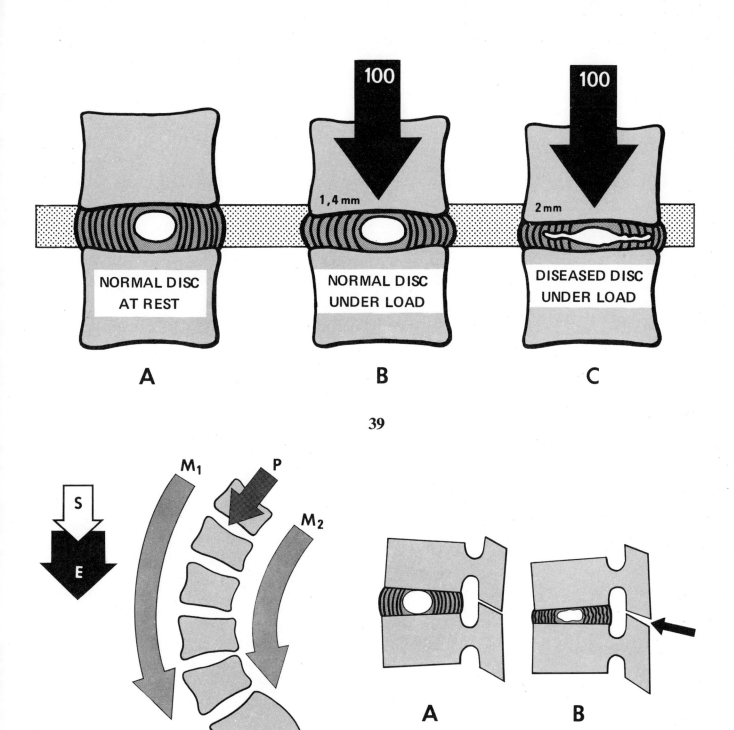

NORMAL DISC
AT REST

A

100

1,4 mm

NORMAL DISC
UNDER LOAD

B

100

2 mm

DISEASED DISC
UNDER LOAD

C

39

M₁

P

S

E

M₂

38

A

B

40

VARIATIONS IN DISC STRUCTURE RELATED TO CORD LEVEL

Disc thickness varies with disc position in the vertebral column (fig. 41). It is thickest **in the lumbar region** (b) amounting to 9 mm; in the thoracic region it is 5 mm thick (a), and in the cervical region 3 mm (c). But more important than its absolute thickness is the ratio of disc thickness to the height of the vertebral body. In fact it is this ratio that accounts for the mobility of the particular segment of the column since *the greater the ratio the greater the mobility*. For instance, the cervical column (c) is the most mobile since it has a ratio disc/body of 2/5; the lumbar column (b) is slightly less mobile with a ratio of 1/3. Finally the thoracic column is the least mobile (a) with a ratio of 1/5.

Sagittal sections of the various segments of the column show that *the nucleus is not exactly in the centre of the disc*. If one divides the antero-posterior thickness of the disc into 10 equal parts then:

in the neck (fig. 42), the nucleus lies at 4/10 thickness from the anterior border and 3/10 from the posterior border, filling in the intermediate 3/10. It lies exactly on the axis of movement (white arrow);

in the thoracic region (fig. 43), the nucleus is equidistant from the anterior and posterior borders of the disc. Once more it amounts to 3/10 of disc thickness but it lies posteriorly to the axis of movement (white arrow, lying anteriorly);

in the lumbar region (fig. 44), the nucleus lies at 4/10 thickness from the anterior border of the disc and 2/10 from the posterior border but it now amounts to 4/10 of disc thickness, i.e., *it has a greater surface area* corresponding to the greater axial forces exerted there. As in the case of the neck region it lies exactly on the axis of movement.

Leonardi considers that the centre of the nucleus is equidistant from the anterior border of the vertebra and the ligamentum flavum. It obviously represents a point of equilibrium, as if the posterior ligaments actively pulled the nucleus posteriorly.

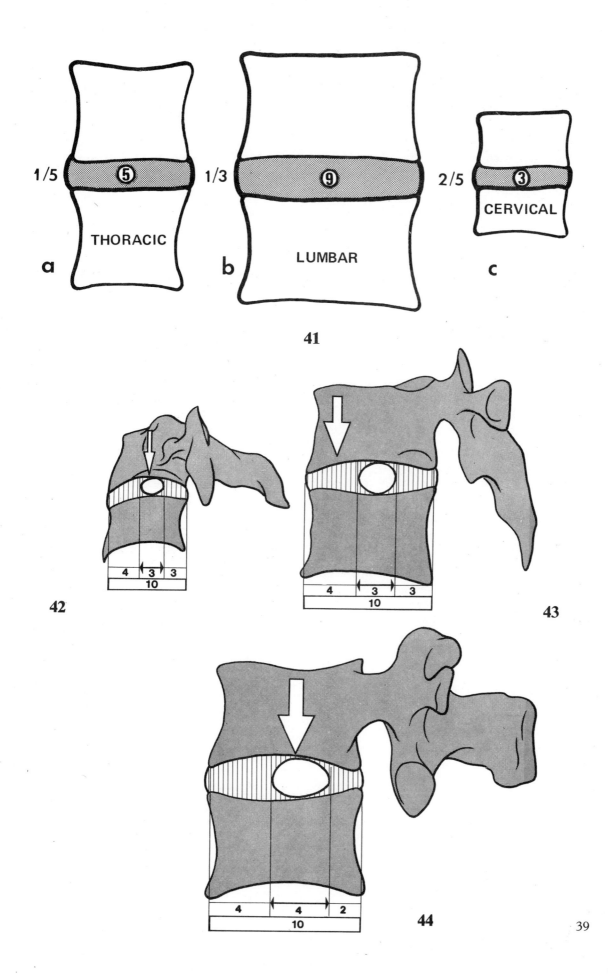

1/5 ⑤ THORACIC

a

1/3 ⑨ LUMBAR

b

2/5 ③ CERVICAL

c

41

4 3 3
10

42

4 3 3
10

43

4 4 2
10

44

39

DISC BEHAVIOUR DURING SIMPLE MOVEMENTS

Let us start with **movements occurring in the axis of the vertebral column** (fig. 45). In the position of rest (A) it has been shown that the fibres of the annulus are already under tension as a result of the *preloaded state of the nucleus.*

When the column is elongated (B) the vertebral bodies tend to move apart increasing the disc height. At the same time its width is reduced while the tension in the annulus fibres rises. The disc, somewhat flattened at rest, now becomes more spherical. This increase in disc height reduces the internal pressure; hence the rationale underlying the treatment of disc prolapse by spinal traction. When the column is elongated the gelatinous substance of the disc moves back into its casing. However, this result is not always achieved because under certain conditions the inner fibres of the annulus may in fact raise the internal pressure of the nucleus.

During axial compression (C) the disc is flattened and widened, the nucleus becomes flatter, raising appreciably its internal pressure, which is transmitted to the innermost fibres of the annulus. Thus a vertical force is transformed into lateral forces tightening up the annular fibres.

Let us now turn to the application of **asymmetrical forces.** *During extension* (fig. 46), the upper vertebra moves posteriorly reducing the interspace posteriorly and driving the nucleus anteriorly. The nucleus presses on the anterior fibres of the annulus increasing their tension and this tends to restore the upper vertebra to its original position.

During flexion (fig. 47), the upper vertebra moves anteriorly reducing the interspace anteriorly and driving the nucleus posteriorly. The nucleus now presses on the posterior fibres of the annulus increasing their tension. Once more one sees the process of self-stabilisation due to the concerted action of the nucleus-annulus couple.

During lateral flexion (fig. 48), the upper vertebra tilts towards the side of flexion and the nucleus is driven to the opposite side. This results in self-stabilisation.

During axial rotation (fig. 49), the oblique fibres, running counter to the direction of movement, are stretched while the intermediate fibres with opposite orientation are relaxed. The tension reaches a maximum in the central fibres of the annulus which are the most oblique. The nucleus is therefore strongly compressed and the internal pressure rises in proportion to the angle of rotation. This explains why flexion and axial rotation tend to tear the annulus and drive the nucleus posteriorly through the tears in the annulus.

When a *static force is applied slightly obliquely to a vertebra* (fig. 50) the vertical force can be resolved into:

a force N perpendicular to inferior vertebral plateau;

a force T parallel to the plateau.

The force N approximates the two vertebrae while the force T makes the upper vertebra slide anteriorly and this leads to a progressive stretching of the oblique fibres in each fibrous layer of the annulus.

On the whole, it is clear that, whatever force is applied to the disc, *it always increases the internal pressure of the disc and stretches the fibres of the annulus.* But, owing to the relative movement of the nucleus, the stretching of the annulus fibres tends to oppose this movement; hence the system tends to be restored to its initial state.

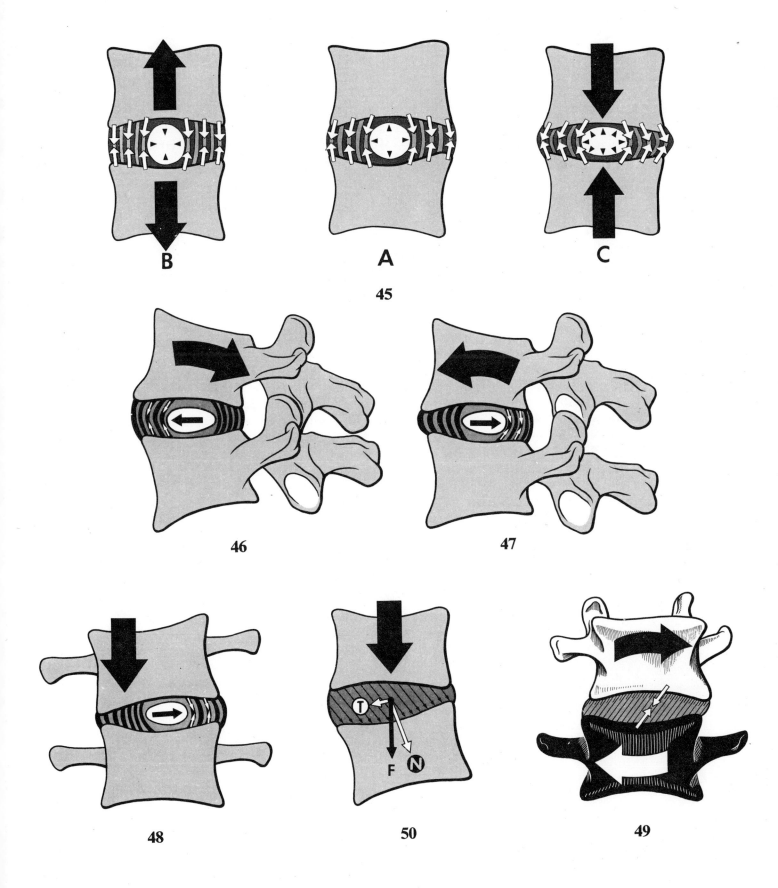

B   A   C

45

46   47

48   50   49

AUTOMATIC ROTATION OF THE VERTEBRAL COLUMN
DURING LATERAL FLEXION

During lateral flexion the vertebral bodies rotate contralaterally. This can be seen on antero-posterior radiograph (fig. 51): the bodies lose their symmetry and the interspinous line (heavy broken line) moves towards the side of movement. In the diagram (fig. 52) a vertebra is accurately drawn so as to allow better understanding of its orientation and of the radiographic findings. When viewed from above (A), the contralateral transverse process appears in full view while the ipsilateral process is foreshortened. Furthermore, in the X-ray film, the interspaces between the contralateral articular processes are seen in succession, while a frontal view is obtained of the ipsilateral articular processes and the pedicles.

This **automatic rotation** of the vertebrae depends on *two mechanisms—compression of intervertebral discs and the stretching of ligaments.* The effect of disc compression is easily displayed on a simple mechanical model (fig. 53). Paste together wedge-shaped segments of cork and soft rubber to represent vertebrae and discs respectively and draw a line centrally on their anterior aspects. If the model is flexed to one side, contralateral rotation of the 'vertebrae' is shown by the displacement of the various segments of the central line. Lateral flexion increases the internal pressure of the 'disc' on the side of movement; as the disc is wedge-shaped its compressed substance tends to escape towards the zone of lower pressure, i.e., contralaterally. This leads to rotation.

This pressure differential is shown in fig. 52A where + marks the high pressure area, and the arrow the direction of rotation.

Conversely, lateral flexion *stretches* the contralateral ligaments, which tend to move towards the midline so as to minimise their lengths. This is shown in fig. 52A as − in relation to an intertransverse ligament and the arrow indicates the direction of movement.

It is remarkable that these two processes are *synergistic* and in their own way contribute to rotation of the vertebrae.

This rotation is normal but in some cases the vertebrae are fixed in a position of rotation as a result of developmental abnormalities and of imbalance of the ligaments. This results in *scoliosis* which combines fixed *lateral flexion* of the column with *rotation* of the vertebrae. This abnormal rotation can be demonstrated clinically (fig. 54). In the normal subject (A), on forward flexion of the trunk the vertebral column is symmetrical posteriorly. If scoliosis is present (B), asymmetry is displayed: the thorax is arched and the vertebral column is bent on the same side of the body. This is due to the *state of fixed rotation of the vertebrae.* Thus the physiological short-lasting automatic rotation of the vertebrae has become pathological in that it is now permanently linked to lateral flexion of the vertebral column.

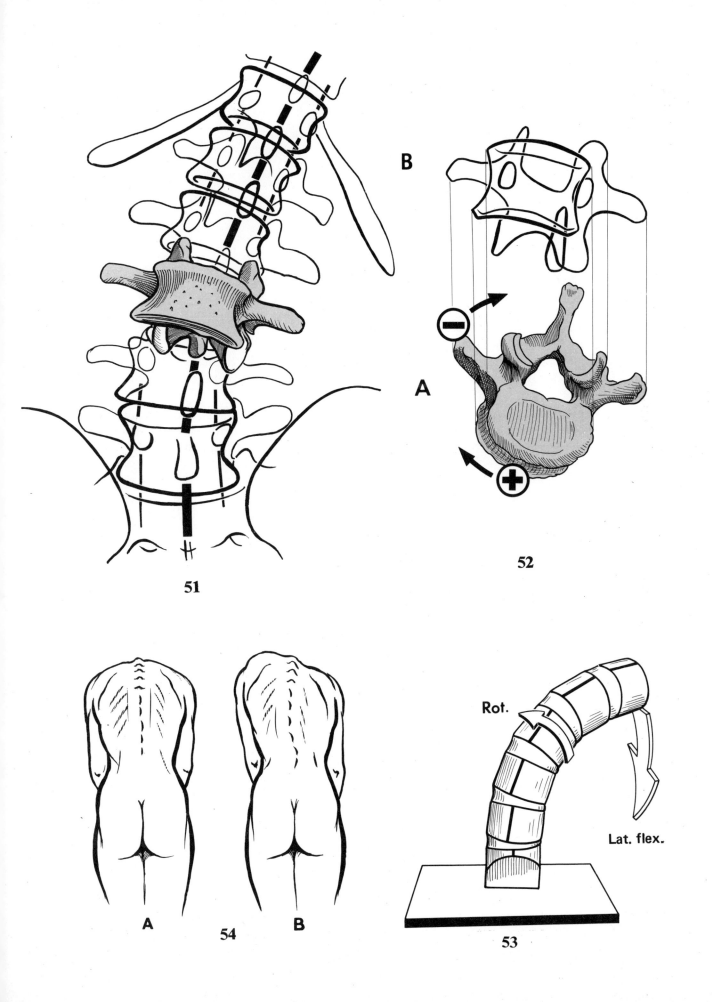

B

51

A

52

Rot.

Lat. flex.

A   54   B

53

FLEXION AND EXTENSION OF THE VERTEBRAL COLUMN: RANGE OF MOVEMENT

As a whole the column from sacrum to skull is equivalent to a joint with *three degrees of freedom*: it allows flexion and extension, lateral flexion right and left and axial rotation. The range of these elementary movements at each individual joint of the column is very small but, in view of the many joints involved, the cumulative effect is quite significant.

Flexion and extension take place in the sagittal plane (fig. 53). The reference plane at skull level is the *plane of the bite*, which can be imagined as a sheet of cardboard tightly held between the teeth. The angle formed by the plane of the bite and the two extreme positions (At) is 250°. This range is considerable when compared to the 180° maximum range of all the other joints of the body. Of course this 250° value applies to the maximum range ever attained in particularly supple individuals.

The *segmental contributions* to this total range can be measured on *oblique radiographs*.

At lumbar level: flexion (Fl) = 60°, extension (El) = 35°.

For the thoraco-lumbar region taken as a whole: flexion (FTL) = 105°, extension (ETL) = 60°.

For the cervical region: flexion (Fc) = 40°; extension (Ec) = 75°.

Therefore the *total range of flexion of the column* (Ft) is 110° and extension is 140°.

These figures are of course approximations as there is no agreement among authors regarding the range of movement at various levels of the column. Moreover these values vary enormously with age. Therefore only maximum values are given here.

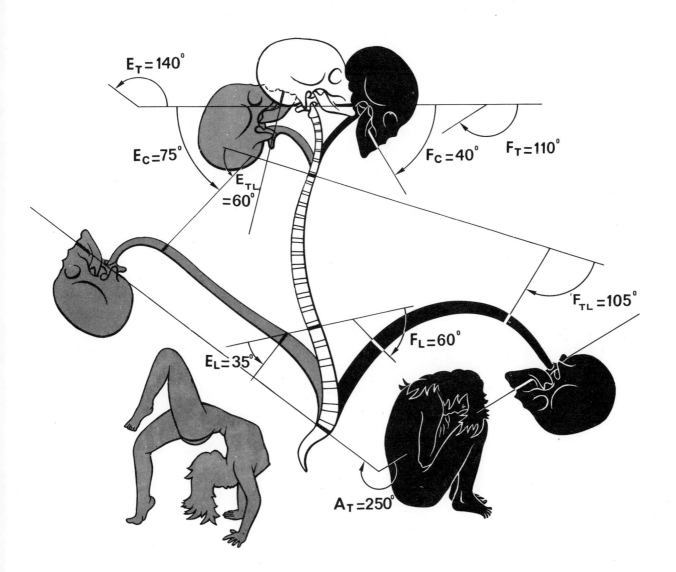

$E_T = 140°$

$E_C = 75°$

$E_{TL} = 60°$

$E_L = 35°$

$F_C = 40°$

$F_T = 110°$

$F_{TL} = 105°$

$F_L = 60°$

$A_T = 250°$

55

RANGE OF LATERAL FLEXION OF THE WHOLE VERTEBRAL COLUMN

Lateral flexion occurs in a *frontal plane* (fig. 56). It is easy to measure these ranges on an antero-posterior radiograph using as reference either the axis of the vertebrae or the orientation of the superior plateau of a particular vertebra. At skull level one can use the intermastoid line, i.e., the line joining the two mastoid processes.

Lateral flexion of the *lumbar column* is 20°.

Lateral flexion of the *thoracic column* is 20°.

Lateral flexion of the *cervical column* is 35°–45°.

Therefore the total range of lateral flexion of the column from sacrum to cranium is 75°–85°.

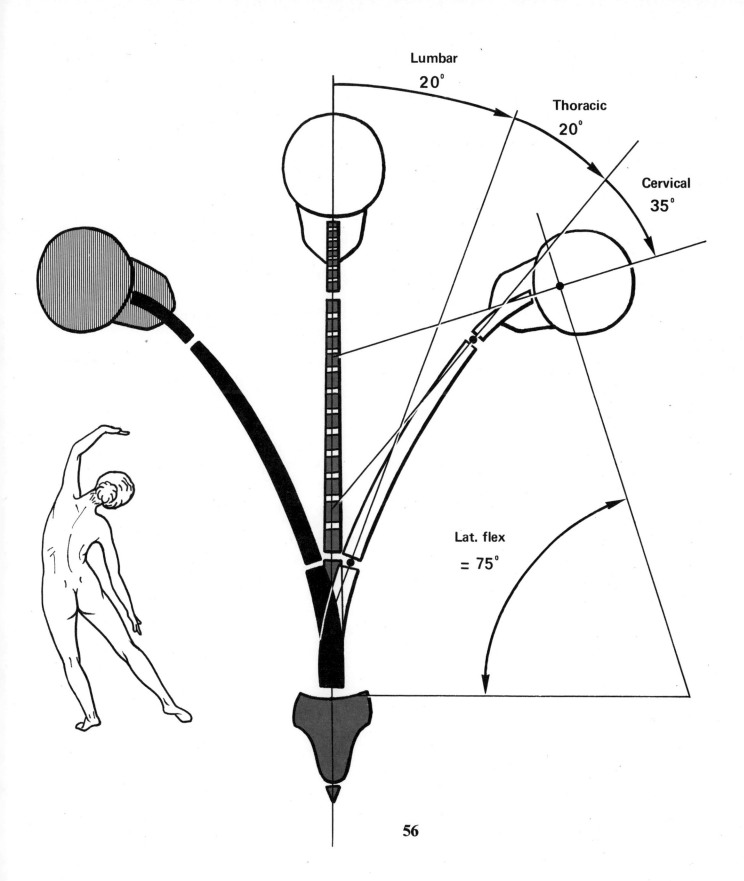

Lumbar
20°

Thoracic
20°

Cervical
35°

Lat. flex
= 75°

56

RANGE OF AXIAL ROTATION OF THE WHOLE VERTEBRAL COLUMN

It is difficult to measure the range of rotation movements, as it is impossible to take radiographs in the transverse plane and axial tomograms lack the definition required to study vertebral rotation. Therefore one can only measure the total rotation of the vertebral column by fixing the pelvis and noting the angle of rotation of the skull.

Recently two American authors (Greggersen and Lucas) have been able to measure accurately the elementary components of rotation by using metal clips, inserted into the spinous processes under anaesthesia. We will come back to this work later.

Axial rotation of the lumbar vertebral column (fig. 57) is very small, only 5°. The reasons for this will become apparent later.

Axial rotation of the *thoracic vertebral column* (fig. 58) is more extensive—35°. It is favoured by the arrangement of the articular processes.

Axial rotation of the *cervical vertebral column* (fig. 59) is quite extensive, attaining 45°–50°. One can see that the atlas has rotated almost 90° with respect to the sacrum.

Axial rotation of the vertebral column *from pelvis to cranium* (fig. 60) attains or exceeds 90°. The atlanto-occipital joint contributes a few degrees of rotation but, as very often the range of rotation in the thoraco-lumbar region is smaller than indicated, total rotation barely attains 90°.

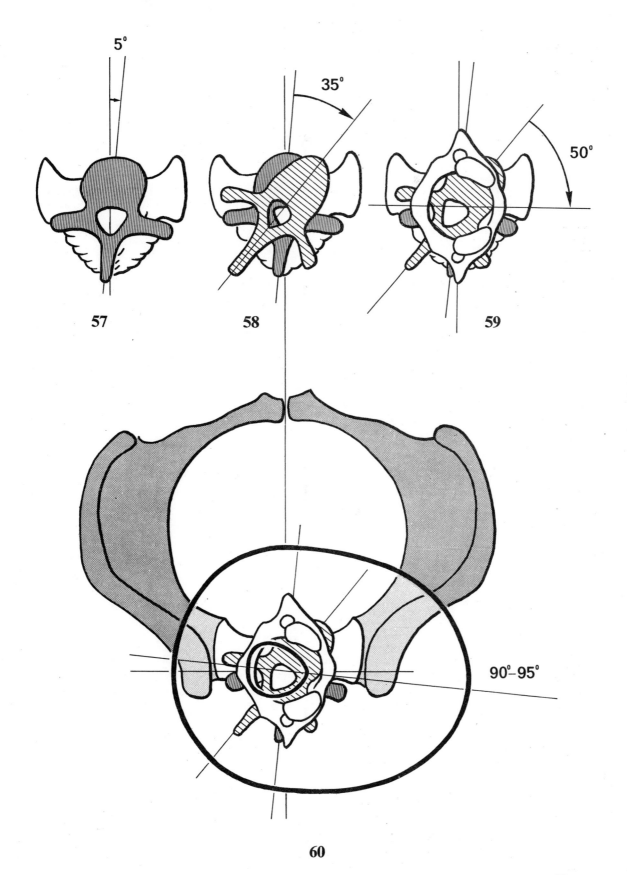

57

58

59

60

CLINICAL ASSESSMENT OF THE RANGE OF MOVEMENTS
OF THE VERTEBRAL COLUMN

Accurate measurements of the range of movements of the vertebral column can only be made radiographically for flexion and extension and lateral flexion.

One can clinically assess the range of movements of the vertebral column by applying certain tests.

To assess *flexion of the thoraco-lumbar column* (fig. 61) one can either:

(a) Measure the **angle** between the vertical and the line joining the antero-superior aspect of the greater trochanter (1) to the angle of the acromion (2). This angle also includes some element of flexion at the hip.

(b) Determine the level of the finger tips (d) during flexion while standing with knees extended; here again some hip flexion is included. One can measure the **distance d** in cm from the fingertips to the ground or the **distance n** from the level of the fingertips to any landmark in the lower limbs, i.e., patella, mid-tibia or toes.

(c) Measure with a tape the distance between the spinous processes of C_7 and S_1 during extension and flexion. In the diagram the distance increases by 5 cm in flexion.

To measure *extension of the thoraco-lumbar column* (fig. 62) one can measure the **angle a** between the vertical and the line joining the antero-superior border of the greater trochanter and the angle of the acromion during maximum extension. This value also includes some degree of extension at the hips. A more accurate method consists of measuring the angle of extension of the vertebral column as a whole (**angle b**) and then subtracting from it the angle of extension of the cervical segment (measured by keeping the trunk vertical and throwing the head backwards). A good test of extension and flexibility of the vertibral column is to 'do the crab' but its usefulness is limited.

To assess *lateral flexion of the thoraco-lumbar vertebral column* (fig. 63), one measures from behind the **angle a** formed between the vertical and the line joining the internatal cleft and the spinous process of C_7. It would be more accurate to measure the **angle b** between the vertical and the tangent to the curve of the vertebral column at C_7. A simpler and quicker method is to determine the **level n** of the fingertips with respect to the knee joint.

To assess *axial rotation* properly one must examine the subject from above (fig. 64). The subject is seated in a low-backed chair and the pelvis is fixed by steadying both the pelvis and the knees. The plane of reference is the frontal plane (F) passing through the vertex of the skull (0). Rotation of the thoraco-lumbar vertebral column is measured as the **angle a** formed between the interscapular line EE′ and the frontal plane.

The range of rotation of the vertebral column as a whole is measured by the angle b, formed between the interauricular line and the frontal plane. One can also measure the angle of rotation (b′) formed between the plane of symmetry of the head (S′) and the sagittal plane (S).

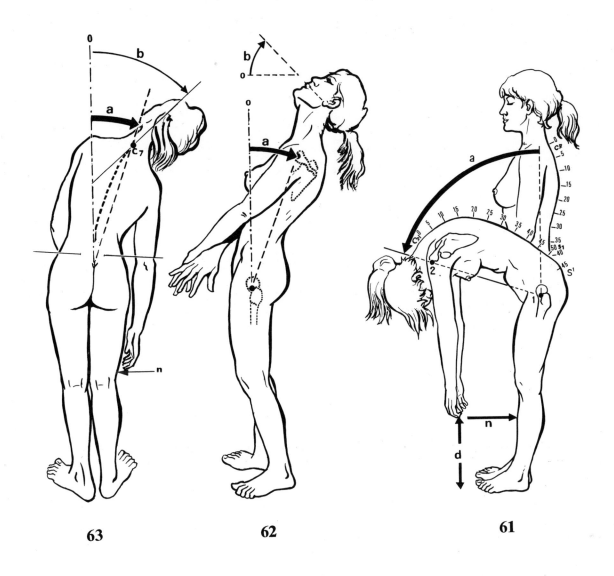

63

62

61

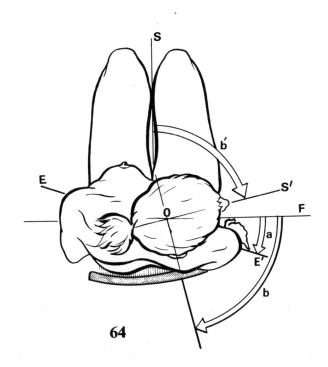

64

51

THE BONY PELVIS AND THE SACRO-ILIAC JOINTS

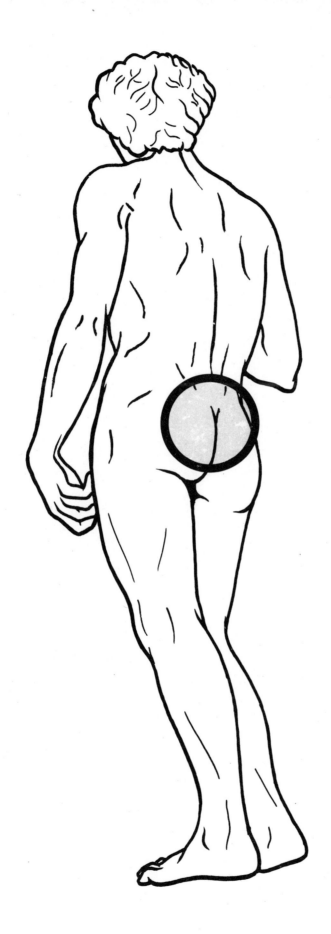

THE BONY PELVIS IN THE TWO SEXES

The bony pelvis constitutes the *base of the trunk*. It supports the abdomen and links the vertebral column to the lower limbs. It is a *closed osteo-articular ring* made up of three bony parts and three joints.

The three bony parts are:

the *two iliac bones*, paired and symmetrical;

the *sacrum*, unpaired but symmetrical, a solid piece of bone resulting from fusion of the five sacral vertebrae.

The three joints are:

the *two sacro-iliac joints* between the sacrum and the iliac bones;

the *symphysis pubis* linking the iliac bones anteriorly.

Taken as a whole the bony pelvis resembles a funnel with the broader base facing superiorly and constituting the pelvic brim that links the abdominal and the pelvic cavities. The bony pelvis is quite different in the two sexes. When one compares the male (fig. 1) and the female (fig. 2) pelves, the latter is seen to be *broader* and more opened out. The triangle containing the female pelvis has a distinctly broader base.

On the other hand, the female pelvis is *shorter* than the male pelvis so that the trapezium containing the female pelvis is lower.

Finally the *pelvic brim* is *larger* and more wide-mouthed in the female.

This structural difference is related to child-bearing since the fetus, especially its relatively large head, lies initially above the pelvis and therefore during labour must cross the pelvic brim before traversing the pelvic cavity. The joints of the bony pelvis therefore are not only important in supporting the erect trunk at rest but also participate in labour, as we shall see in discussing the physiology of the sacro-iliac joint.

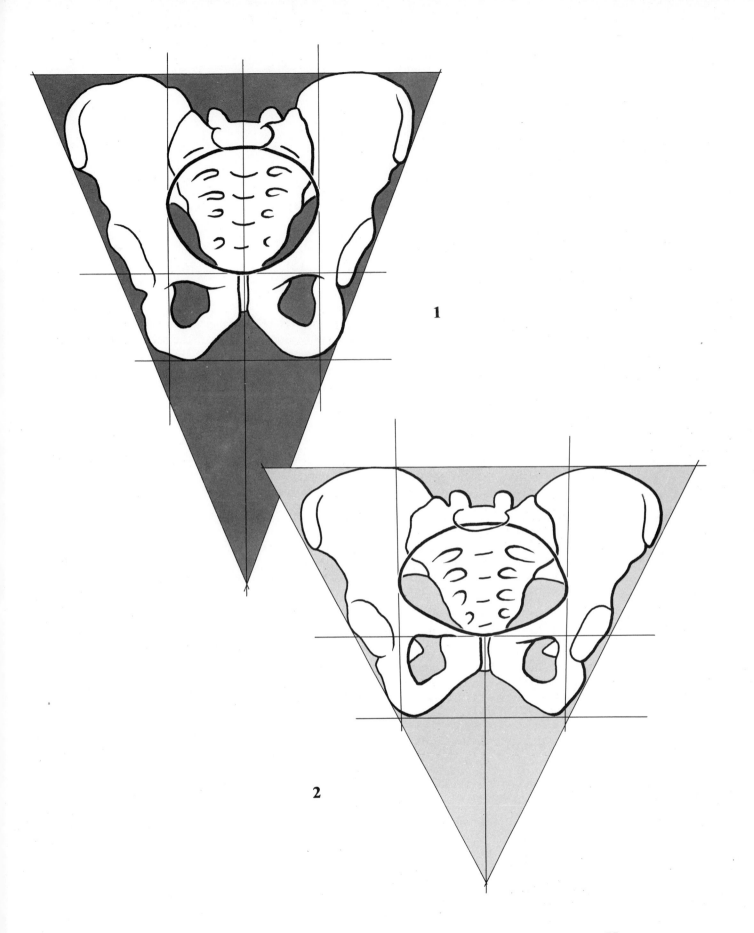

1

2

55

STRUCTURE OF THE BONY PELVIS

As a whole the bony pelvis *transmits forces from the vertebral column to the lower limbs* (fig. 3). The weight (P) supported by L5 is distributed equally along the alae of the sacrum and through the ischial tuberosities towards the acetabulum. Part of the reaction of the ground to the body weight (R) is transmitted to the acetabulum by the neck and head of the femur. The rest is transmitted across the horizontal ramus of the pubic bone and is counterbalanced at the symphysis pubis by a similar force from the other side.

These lines of force form a **complete ring** along the pelvic brim. There is a *complex system of bony trabeculae in the pelvic bones corresponding to the lines of force* (see vol. II, page 28).

As the sacrum is broader above than below it can be taken as a wedge (dark hatched triangle) which fits vertically between the two iliac bones. The sacrum is suspended from these bones by ligaments and so it is the more tightly held the heavier the weight it is bearing. It is therefore a *self-locking system*.

The sacrum also fits between the iliac bones in the *transverse plane* (figs. 4 and 5). Each iliac bone can be taken as a lever arm (fig. 4) with its fulcrum located at the sacro-iliac joint. Its mechanical resistance resides posteriorly in the powerful sacro-iliac ligaments (L1 and L2), while its power is expressed anteriorly at the *pubic symphysis* where two approximating forces are acting (S1 and S2).

If the **pubic symphysis is dislocated** (fig. 5), the separation of the two pubic bones (S) leads to a wider spacing of the iliac bones so that the sacrum, being less tightly held, can move forward (d_1 and d_2).

One can thus understand the *complete interdependence of the various elements of the pelvic brim* so that any impairment at any level affects the structure as a whole and decreases its mechanical resistance.

P

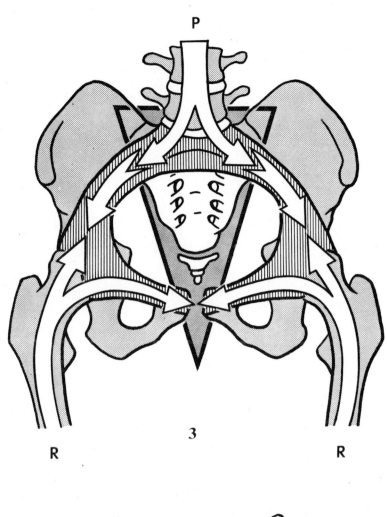

3

R R

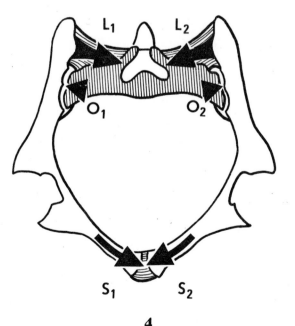

L₁ L₂

O₁ O₂

S₁ S₂

4

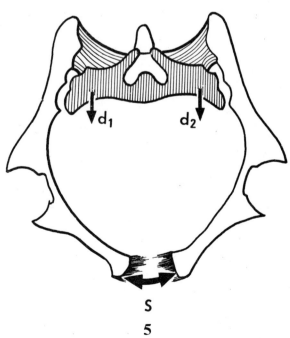

d₁ d₂

S

5

57

THE ARTICULAR SURFACES OF THE SACRO-ILIAC JOINT

If one opens the sacro-iliac joint (fig. 6) like a book by swivelling the two bony elements about a vertical axis (a, b, c) *the articular surfaces are clearly seen to be corresponding*:

the articular surface of the iliac bone (A) lying on the postero-superior part of the medial aspect of the iliac bone, just posterior to the ilio-pectineal line, which forms part of the pelvic brim. It is crescent-shaped, concave postero-superiorly and is lined by cartilage. As a whole the surface is pretty irregular but Farabeuf has compared it to a segment of rail. In fact its long axis contains a long crest lying between two furrows. This curved crest corresponds to an arc of a circle whose centre lies approximately at the sacral tuberosity (black cross). As we shall see, this tuberosity is the point of insertion of the powerful sacro-iliac ligaments;

the articular surface of the sacrum (B) which corresponds in shape and surface to the articular surface of the iliac bone. In the centre there is a curved furrow bordered by two long crests and corresponding to an arc of a circle whose centre lies on the transverse tubercle of S_1 (black cross). This tubercle is the point of insertion of some powerful ligaments of the sacro-iliac joint. Farabeuf has compared this surface to a *tram-rail*, corresponding exactly to the rail-like surface of the iliac bone.

However, these two surfaces are not as regular as described above and three horizontal sections (fig. 7) taken at levels a, b and c of fig. 6 show that only in its middle (b) and superior (a) portions does the sacral articular facet bear a central furrow. Its inferior portion (c) is more or less convex centrally. As a result, it is difficult to demonstrate the whole interspace of the sacro-iliac joint in a single radiograph. Multiple exposures are required to study the various segments of the joint.

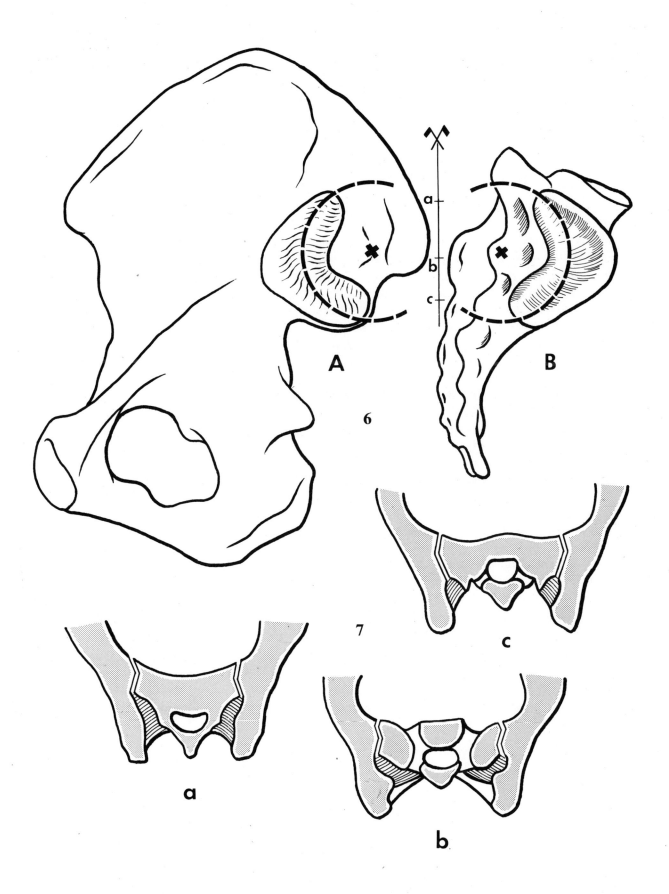

A   B

6

7

a

b

c

THE ARTICULAR FACET OF THE SACRUM

The sacral articular facet is subject to **wide structural variations** from person to person, and A. Delmas has demonstrated a *correlation between the functional type of vertebral column and the structure of the sacrum and its articular facet* (fig. 8).

When the *curvatures of the vertebral column are pronounced* (A)—*the dynamic type*—the sacrum lies horizontally and its articular facet is at once markedly buckled on itself and deep. The sacro-iliac joint is highly mobile resembling the typical synovial joints and its represents an example of overadaptation to the biped state.

When the *curvatures of the vertebral column are poorly developed* (B)—*the static type*—the sacrum is almost vertical and its articular facet is elongated vertically, slightly buckled on itself and almost flat. This structural constitution of the articular facet is quite different from the one described by Farabeuf and corresponds to a joint of low mobility, like the secondary cartilaginous joints. It is often seen in children and closely resembles that found in the primates.

A. Delmas has shown that during evolution from primates to man the caudal segment of the articular facet becomes longer and longer and assumes in man greater significance than the cranial segment. In man the angle between these two segments can attain 90° while in primates the articular facet is only minimally buckled.

The **surface contours** of the sacral articular facet have been studied in detail by Weisel who has shown (fig. 9) that the cranial segment of the sacral articular facet is usually longer and narrower than its caudal counterpart. The sacral facet shows regularly a central depression at the junction of its two segments (shown as −) and two elevations near the edges of these two segments (shown as +). The iliac facet is reciprocally structured but without complete correspondence. At the junction of the two segments of the iliac articular facet there is a slight elevation known as Bonnaire's tubercle.

Weisel has also developed a personal theory regarding the *distribution of the sacro-iliac ligaments* in terms of the applied forces. He divides these ligaments into two groups (fig. 10):

a cranial group (Cr), running laterally and posteriorly and counteracting the component F_1 of the body weight P, which is applied to the superior aspect of S_1. These ligaments are thrown into action by forward displacement of the sacral promontory;

a caudal group (Ca), running craniad and counteracting the component F_2, acting perpendicularly to the superior surface of S_1.

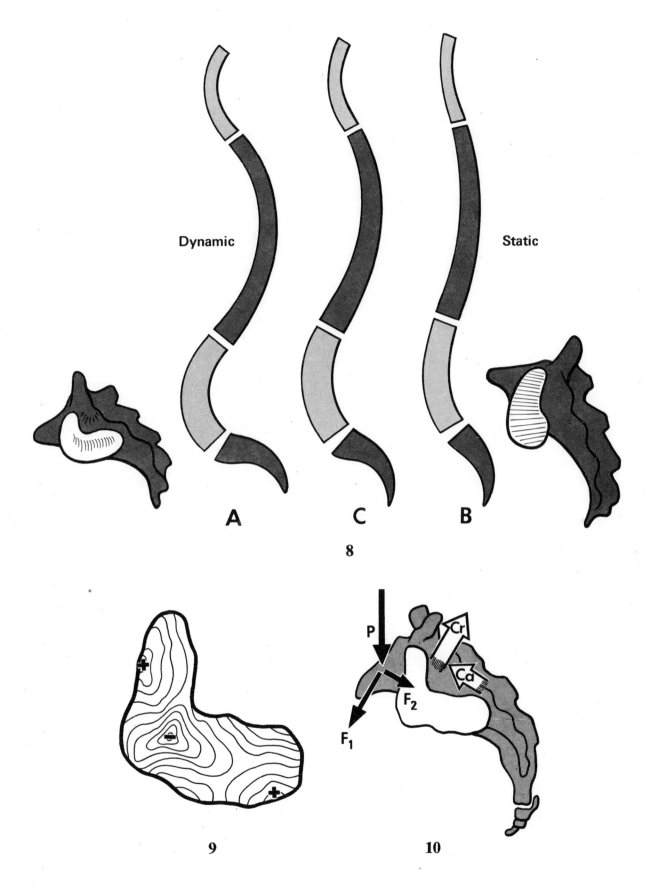

Dynamic

Static

A   C   B

8

9

10

THE SACRO-ILIAC LIGAMENTS

(The numbers have the same meaning in all three diagrams.)

A posterior view of the pelvis (fig. 11) shows the following:

A The iliolumbar ligaments

the *superior band* of the iliolumbar ligament (1);

the *inferior band* of the iliolumbar ligament (2).

B The intermediate plane of the sacro-iliac ligaments on the right side:

the ligament running from the iliac crest to the transverse tubercle of S_1 (3).

the four ligaments running from the posterior aspect of the iliac crest to the sacral tubercles (4), as described by Farabeuf: the first running from the iliac crest to the tubercle of S_1; the second (the ligament of Zaglas) inserting into the tubercle of S_2; the third and fourth running from the postero-superior aspect of the iliac crest to the tubercles of S_3 and S_4.

C The anterior plane of the sacro-iliac ligaments (5) on the left side:

it consists of a fibrous band running from the posterior edge of the iliac bone to the articular tubercles of the sacrum.

D The sacrospinous and sacrotuberous ligaments:

the *sacrospinous ligament* (6), which runs obliquely from the ischial spine to the lateral border of the sacrum and coccyx. It is directed superiorly, medially and posteriorly;

the *sacrotuberous ligament* (7) crosses obliquely the posterior aspect of the former. Superiorly it is attached along a line running from the posterior border of the iliac bone to the first two vertebrae of the coccyx. Its oblique fibres run a twisting course inferiorly, anteriorly and laterally to be inserted into the inferior aspect of the ischial tuberosity and the medial lip of the ascending ramus of the ischium. The sciatic notch is thus divided by these two ligaments into two openings: the *greater sciatic foramen superiorly*, which allows exit of the *piriformis muscle*; the *lesser sciatic foramen inferiorly* which transmits the tendon of the obturator internus.

An anterior view of the pelvis (fig. 12) shows again the iliolumbar (1 and 2), the sacrospinous (6) and the sacrotuberous ligaments (7) and in addition the **anterior sacro-iliac ligament** consisting of two bands: *antero-superior* (8) and *antero-inferior* (9).

Fig. 13 shows the right sacro-iliac joint, opened by rotation of the constituent bones about a vertical axis, and its ligaments. The medial surface of the iliac bone (A) and the lateral surface (B) of the sacrum are exposed. One can see:

how the ligaments are *wrapped around the joint* and how they become lax or taut;

that the *fibres of the anterior sacro-iliac ligament* (8 and 9) run an oblique course from the iliac bone (A) inferiorly, anteriorly and medially. From the sacrum (B) they run an oblique course superiorly, anteriorly and laterally;

the *intermediate sacro-iliac ligaments* (5);

the *sacrospinous* (6) and *sacrotuberous ligaments* (7);

the short axial ligament (shown as a white slice in both diagrams) constitutes the deep layer of the sacro-iliac ligaments and is attached laterally to the lateral aspect of the posterior superior iliac spine and medially to the anterior foramina S_1 and S_2. It is also known as the interosseous ligament and is classically considered to represent the axis of movement of the sacrum—hence the name axial.

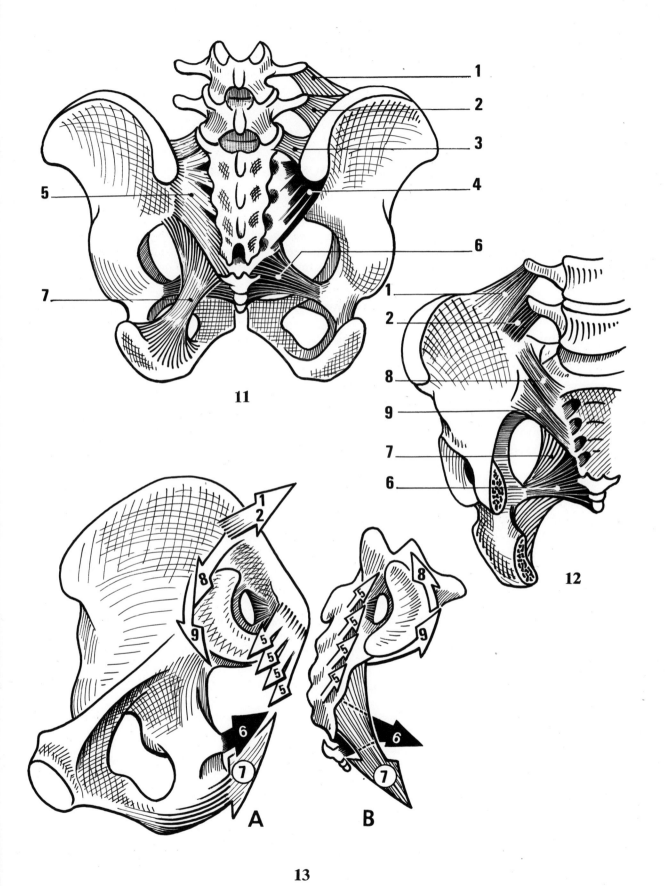

11

12

13

63

NUTATION AND COUNTER-NUTATION

Before studying the movements at the sacro-iliac joint it is wise to recall that their range is small and *varies according to circumstances and the subject*, which explains the lack of agreement regarding the function of this joint and the relevance of its movements during labour. These movements were first described by Zaglas in 1851 and by Duncan in 1854.

The Classical Theory of Nutation and Counter-Nutation

During the movement of nutation (fig. 15) the sacrum rotates about an axis constituted by the axial ligament (shown as a cross) so that the promontory moves inferiorly and anteriorly (S_2), while the apex of the sacrum and the tip of the coccyx move posteriorly (d_2). Thus the antero-posterior diameter of the pelvic brim is reduced by a distance S_2 while the antero-posterior diameter of the pelvic outlet is increased by a distance d_2. Meanwhile (fig. 16), the iliac bones are approximated whereas the ischial tuberosities move apart. The movement of nutation (fig. 13) is limited by the tension developed in the sacrotuberous (7) and sacrospinous (6) ligaments as well as the anterosuperior (8) and anteroinferior (9) bands of the anterior sacro-iliac ligament.

The movement of counter-nutation (fig. 14) involves displacements in the opposite direction. The sacrum, pivoting around the axial ligament, rights itself so that the promontory moves superiorly and posteriorly (S_1) and the apex of the sacrum and the tip of the coccyx move inferiorly and anteriorly (d_1). As a result the anteroposterior diameter of the pelvic brim is increased by a distance S_1 while that of the pelvic outlet is reduced by a distance d_1. Also the iliac bones move apart and the ischial tuberosities are drawn together. The movement of counter-nutation (fig. 13) is limited by the tension developed in the sacro-iliac ligaments both in the anterior (5) and posterior (4) planes.

For example, the change in the anteroposterior diameter of the pelvic brim amounts to 3 mm according to Bonnaire, Pinard and Pinzani, and to 8–13 mm according to Walcher. The change in the anteroposterior diameter of the pelvic outlet can amount to 15 mm according to Borcel and Fernström and 17.5 mm according to Thoms. The lateral displacement of the iliac bones and ischial tuberosities has recently been confirmed by Weisel.

Nutation (Lat. **nutare** = to nod) describes a complex movement of the sacrum analogous to nodding of the head.

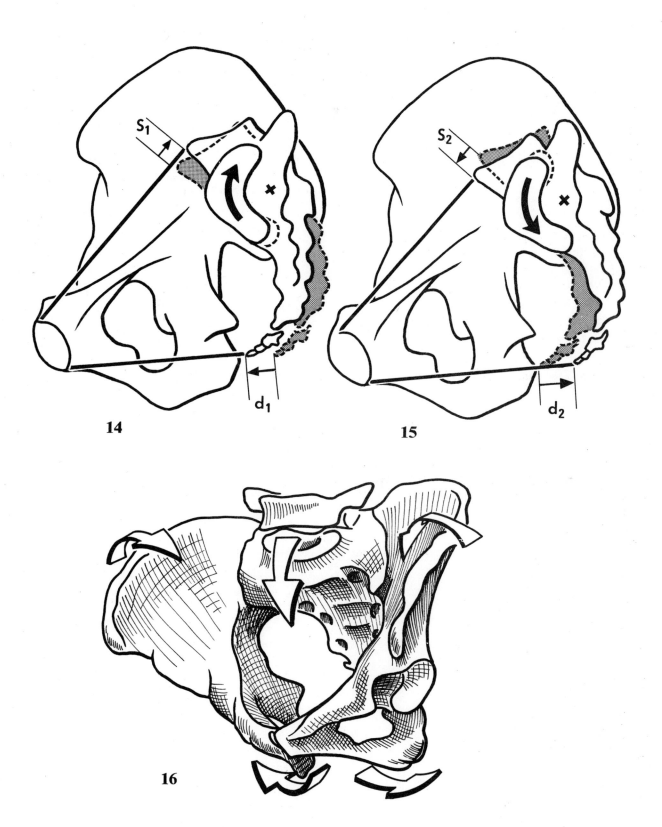

14

15

16

THE VARIOUS THEORIES OF NUTATION

According to the classical theory of Farabeuf (fig. 17), which we have just described, the tilting of the sacrum occurs about an axis constituted by the *axial ligament* (O), its displacement is *angular* and the promontory moves inferiorly and anteriorly along the arc of circle with centre O located posterior to the articular facet.

According to Bonnaire's theory (fig. 18), the tilting of the sacrum occurs about an axis O′, which passes through Bonnaire's tubercle located between the cranial and caudal segments of the sacral articular facet. Therefore the centre of this angular displacement of the sacrum lies within the articular facet.

The studies of Weisel allow two other possible theories:

the theory of pure linear displacement (fig. 19), stating that the sacrum slides along the axis of the caudal portion of the articular facet. This would mean a **linear displacement d** of the sacrum resulting in a corresponding displacement of the sacral promontory and apex.

another theory based on rotational movement (fig. 20):

Here the axis O″ lies anterior to the articular facet and inferior and anterior to the sacrum. The position of this centre would vary from person to person and with the type of movement carried out.

The number of theories available suggests how difficult it is to analyse movements of small range and raises the possibility that different types of movement may occur in different individuals.

These ideas do not merely have abstract significance since these movements participate in the physiology of labour.

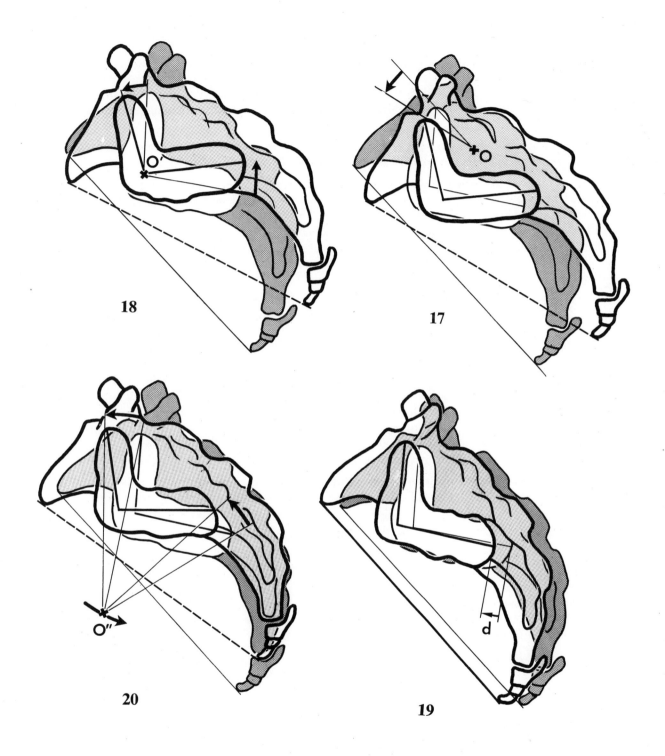

18

17

20

19

THE PUBIC SYMPHYSIS AND THE SACRO-COCCYGEAL JOINT

The **pubic symphysis** is a *secondary cartilaginous joint (amphiarthrosis)* of *minimal mobility*, if any at all. However, near term and during labour water imbibition by its soft tissues allows the two pubic bones to slide on each other and move apart. In rodents these movements have a sizeable range.

The **horizontal section** (fig. 21) shows the two ends of the pubic bones lined axially by cartilage and joined by a fibro-cartilaginous disc—the *interosseous ligament*.

Looking at the joint from inside (fig. 22), the articular surface of the pubic bone is oval with its oblique long axis running superiorly and anteriorly and gives insertion to the rectus abdominis (1). The joint is closed anteriorly by the very thick *anterior ligament* (3), made up of transverse and oblique fibres as seen in an anterior view (fig. 28). The aponeurotic expansions from the transversus abdominis (8), the rectus abdominis (7), the pyramidalis (2), the internal obliquus abdominis and the adductor longus (9) crisscross anterior to the symphysis and form a dense feltwork of fibres.

The posterior aspect of the joint (fig. 24) bears the *posterior ligament* (5) which is a fibrous membrane continuous with the periosteum. **A vertical section taken in a frontal plane** (fig. 23) shows the structure of the articular surfaces *lined by hyaline cartilage* (10), the fibro-cartilaginous disc (11) and its thin central cleft (12). The superior aspect of the joint is strengthened by the *superior ligament* (6) which is a thick and dense fibrous band. The inferior border of the joint is strengthened by the *inferior ligament* (4) or the subpubic arched ligament, which is continuous with the interosseous ligament and forms a sharp-edged arcade rounding off the apex of the pubic arch. The thickness and strength of this ligament can be seen in a sagittal section (fig. 22). These strong periarticular ligaments make the symphysis a strong joint which is not easily dislocated. In clinical practice dislocation rarely occurs and in general when it occurs it is difficult to treat, which is surprising for a joint which is fixed normally.

The **sacro-coccygeal joint**, connecting the sacrum and coccyx, is also a *secondary cartilaginous joint* (amphiarthrosis). Its articular surfaces are elliptical with their long axes lying transversely.

A lateral view (fig. 28) shows the sacral articular surface to be convex and the coccygeal surface concave. The joint is united by an *interosseous ligament* similar to an intervertebral disc and by external ligaments which fall into three groups: anterior, posterior and lateral.

An anterior view (fig. 26) shows the coccyx (1) which is made up of four fused bony vertebrae, the sacrum (2) and the *anterior ligament*. On the anterior aspect of the sacrum, the ends of the anterior longitudinal vertebral ligament (3) become continuous with the anterior sacro-coccygeal ligament (4). Three lateral *sacro-coccygeal ligaments* (5, 6, 7) can also be seen.

A posterior view (fig. 27) shows the end of the posterior longitudinal ligament overlying the superior aspect of the sacrum (8) and becoming continuous with the *posterior sacro-coccygeal ligaments* (9).

The sacro-coccygeal joint exhibits only *flexion and extension* which are essentially *passive* and occur during defecation and labour. In fact during the movement of nutation of the sacrum the posterior tilting of the tip of the sacrum can be amplified and prolonged by extension of the coccyx (i.e., inferiorly and posteriorly). This increases the anteroposterior diameter of the pelvic outlet during delivery of the fetal head.

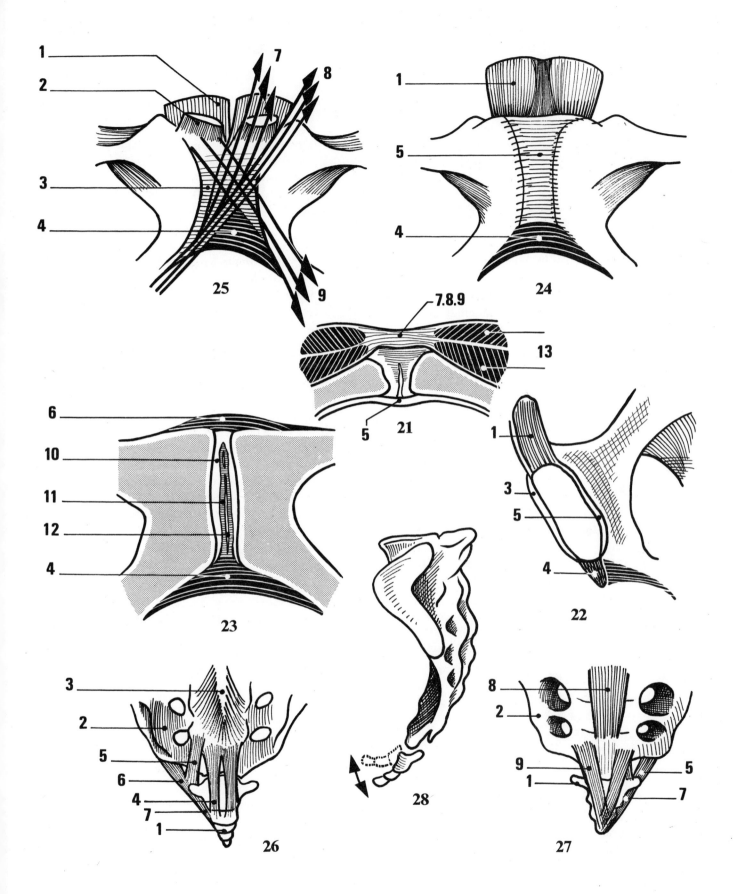

25

7
8
9

1
2

3
4

24

1

5

4

7.8.9

13

5
21

23

6

10

11
12

4

22

1

3

5

4

26

3

2

5
6
4
7
1

28

27

8

2

9
1

5

7

69

EFFECT OF POSTURE ON THE JOINTS OF THE BONY PELVIS

When one stands at ease the joints of the bony pelvis are called into action by the body weight. The mode of action of these forces can be analysed (fig. 29) on a lateral view of the pelvis with the iliac bone considered transparent so that the femur can be seen. The vertebral column, the sacrum, the iliac bone and the lower limbs form a *co-ordinated articular system* with two joints, i.e., the hip joint and the sacro-iliac joint. The *weight of the trunk* (arrow P), acting on the superior surface of S_1, tends to lower the promontory. The sacrum is then induced to rotate, i.e., there occurs a movement of nutation (N_1). This movement is rapidly limited by the anterior sacro-iliac ligaments, and especially by the sacrospinous and sacrotuberous ligaments, which stop the tip of the sacrum moving away from the ischial tuberosity.

At the same time, the *reaction of the ground* (arrow R), transmitted by the femora and applied to the hips, forms with the body weight a *rotatory couple* which, acting at the sacrum, causes the iliac bone to tilt posteriorly (arrow N_2). This backward tilt of the pelvis accentuates the movement of nutation occurring at the sacro-iliac joints.

This analysis, though it deals with movements, should rather deal with forces as in fact movements scarcely occur. There is more a tendency to movement than actual movement since the extremely powerful ligaments preclude any movement from the start.

When one stands on one foot (fig. 30) and when one takes a step during walking, the reaction of the ground (arrow R), transmitted by the supporting limb, elevates the corresponding hip while the contralateral hip tends to be pulled down by the weight of the free limb. This leads to a *shearing force* at the level of the pubic symphysis which tends to raise the hip on the supporting side (A) and lower the contralateral hip (B). Normally the strength of the symphysis precludes any movement but, if it is dislocated, a displacement d can be seen above the symphysis during walking. In the same way, one can imagine that the sacro-iliac joints are mobilised in opposite fashion during walking. Their resistance to movements resides in their strong ligaments but, following traumatic damage to one of the sacro-iliac joints, movements occur and pain is felt at every step. Therefore both standing and walking depend on the mechanical strength of the bony pelvis.

When one lies down, the sacro-iliac joints are called into action in a different way (fig. 33) depending on whether the hip is flexed (A) or extended (B).

When the hips are extended (fig. 32), the traction on the flexor muscles (white arrow) causes the pelvis to tilt anteriorly while the tip of the sacrum is pushed anteriorly. This shortens the distance between the sacral tip and the ischial tuberosity and leads simultaneously to a rotation at the sacro-iliac joint, i.e., *a movement of counternutation* (arrow 2 indicates the movement of the iliac bone about the axis of nutation). This position corresponds to *the early stage of labour* and the counter-nutation, which enlarges the pelvic brim, *favours the descent of the fetal head* into the pelvis.

When the hips are flexed (fig. 31), the traction on the hamstrings (arrow) tends to tilt the pelvis posteriorly relative to the sacrum. This is therefore a *movement of nutation* (the arrow 1 indicates the movement of the iliac bone relative to the sacrum), which decreases the antero-posterior diameter of the pelvic brim and increases both diameters of the pelvic outlet. This position, taken during the *expulsive phase of labour, favours therefore the delivery of the fetal head* as it traverses the pelvic outlet.

During a change of position from hip extension to hip flexion, the mean range of displacement of the promontory is 5.6 mm. Therefore these changes in the position of the thighs markedly alter the dimensions of the pelvic cavity and facilitate the passage of the fetal head during labour.

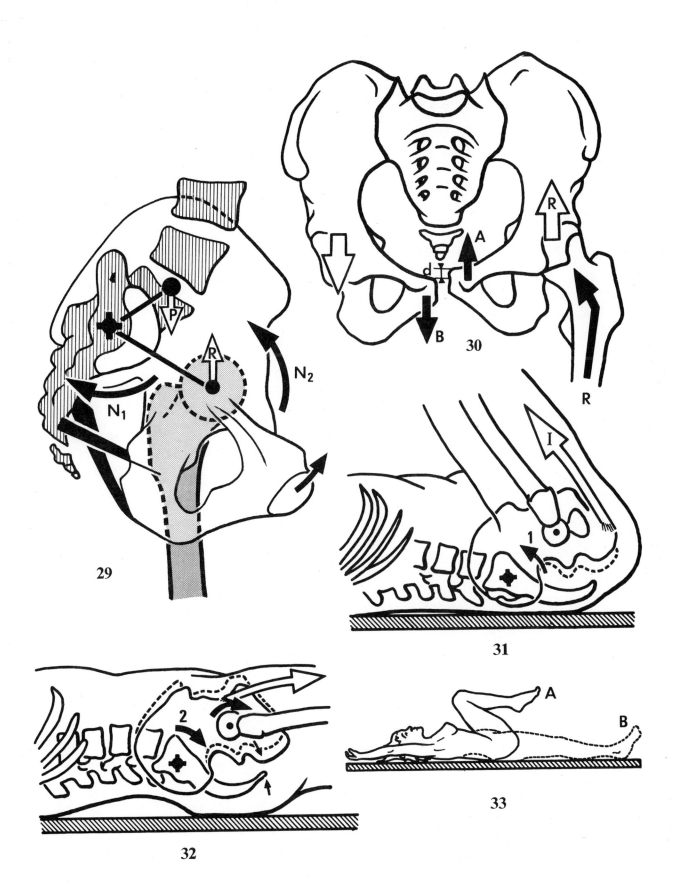

29

30

31

32

33

THE LUMBAR VERTEBRAL COLUMN

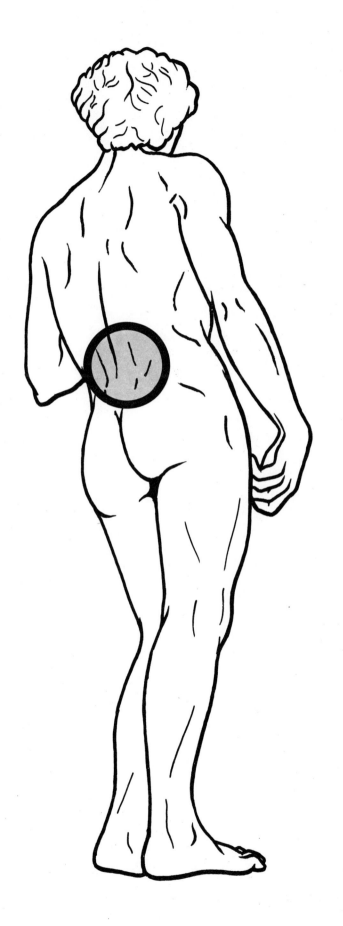

THE LUMBAR VERTEBRAL COLUMN VIEWED AS A WHOLE

When seen on an anteroposterior radiograph (fig. 1) the lumbar column is *straight and symmetrical* relative to the interspinous line (m). The width of the vertebral bodies and of the transverse processes regularly decrease craniad. The horizontal line (h), passing through the highest point of the iliac crests, runs between L_4 and L_5. The vertical lines (a and a′) drawn along the lateral border of the sacral alae run approximately through the acetabula.

An oblique view (fig. 2) shows the features of the *lumbar lordosis and of the lumbar vertebral column at rest*, as worked out by De Seze:

the angle of the sacrum (a), formed between the horizontal and the line running through the superior aspect of S_1, averages 30°;

the lumbosacral angle (b), lying between the axis of L_5 and the sacral axis, averages 140°;

the angle of pelvic tilt (c), formed by the horizontal and the line joining the promontory to the superior border of the pubic symphysis, averages 60°;

the index of lumbar lordosis (white arrow f) can be determined by joining the superoposterior border of L_1 to the posteroinferior border of L_5. The perpendicular to this line is usually maximal at L_3 and represents the *index of lordosis*. It is greater as lordosis is more marked and almost disappears when the column is straight. It can rarely become inverted.

the posterior projection (white arrow r) represents the distance between the posteroinferior border of L_5 and the vertical line passing through the posteroinferior border of L_1. It can be *positive* if the lumbar column is thrown backwards; it can be negative if the column is *flexed*.

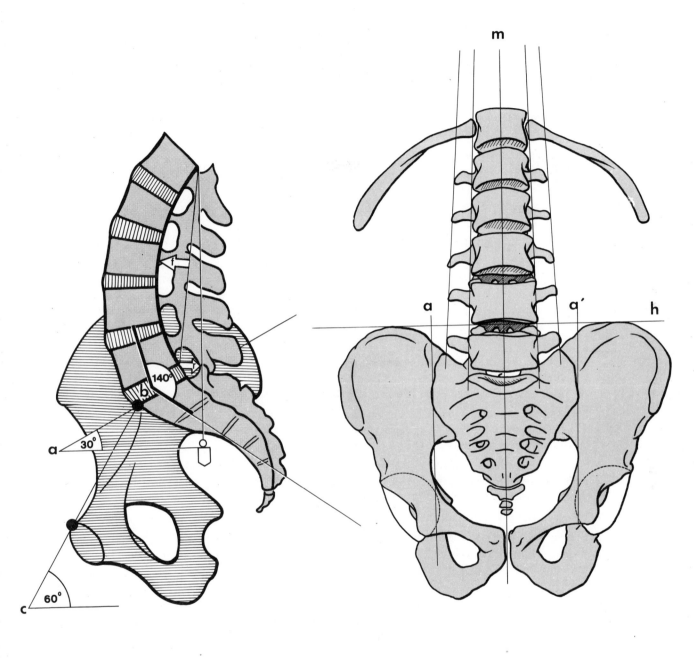

2

1

STRUCTURE OF LUMBAR VERTEBRAE

If a lumbar vertebra is viewed from the back (fig. 4) its constituents are seen as follows (fig. 3: vertebra 'exploded'):

the kidney-shaped vertebral body (1) is wider laterally than it is deep anteroposteriorly; and broader than it is high. Its periphery is deeply hollowed out in the shape of a diabolo, except posteriorly where it is nearly flat;

the two laminae (2) are highly set and run posteriorly and medially but they lie in a plane which is oblique inferiorly and laterally;

the laminae meet in the midline to form a *spinous process* (3) which is quite large and rectangular, points posteriorly and has a bulbous posterior tip;

the *transverse processes* (4), better called costoid processes since they are in fact rib vestiges. They are attached at the level of the articular processes and run an oblique course posteriorly and laterally. On the posterior aspect of the site of attachment of these transverse processes lies the accessory process which, according to some authors, is the homologue of the transverse process of the thoracic vertebra;

the pedicle (5), a short bony segment joining the vertebral body to the vertebral arch and attached to the former at its superolateral angle. It constitutes the superior and inferior limits of the intervertebral foramen and posteriorly it provides attachment for the articular processes;

the superior articular process (6) lies on the superior border of the lamina as it joins the pedicle. It lies in a plane oblique posteriorly and laterally and its cartilage-lined articular surface faces posteriorly and medially;

the inferior articular process (7) arises from the inferior border of the vertebral arch near the junction of the lamina with the spinous process. It faces inferiorly and medially and its cartilage-lined articular surface faces laterally and anteriorly;

between the posterior surface of the vertebral body and the vertebral arch is the *vertebral canal* in the shape of an almost equilateral triangle.

Some lumbar vertebrae have *certain peculiarities*, e.g., the transverse process of L is less well developed than that of the other lumbar vertebrae.

The *vertebral body of* L_5 is higher anteriorly than posteriorly so that its profile is *wedge-shaped* or even trapezoidal with its longer side lying anteriorly. Its articular processes are more widely separated from each other than with the other lumbar vertebrae.

When two lumbar vertebrae are separated (fig. 5A) one sees how the inferior articular processes of the upper vertebra fit medially and posteriorly into the superior articular processes of the lower vertebra (fig. 5B). Therefore each lumbar vertebra stabilises laterally the overlying vertebra as a result of the buttress-like structure of the articular processes.

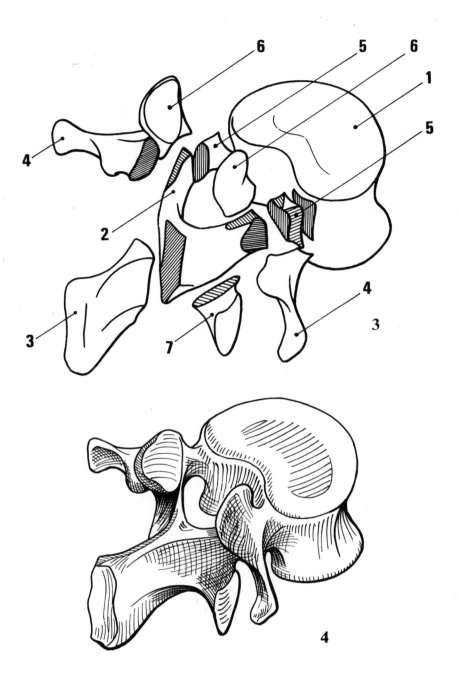

4

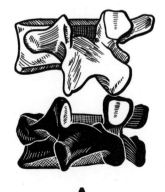

A

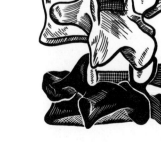

B

5

THE LIGAMENTS OF THE LUMBAR VERTEBRAL COLUMN

The ligaments can be studied, on the one hand, on a *sagittal section* (fig. 6) after removal of the laminae on the left and, on the other, on a frontal section (fig. 7) taken through the pedicles. The anterior half of the section containing the vertebral bodies is seen from behind and the posterior half of the section, after having been rotated 180°, contains the vertebral arches seen from the front (fig. 8). A detached vertebra is also seen above. Note that in figs. 7 and 8 one sees the corresponding stumps of the pedicles. (The same numbers apply to all three diagrams.)

In the sagittal section (fig. 6) can be seen **two sets of ligaments**:

on the one hand, running all along the vertebral column, the *anterior* (1) *and posterior* (5) *longitudinal ligaments*;

on the other hand, *segmental ligaments* running between vertebral arches.

The anterior longitudinal ligament (1) stretches as a long dense band from the basi-occiput to the sacrum on the anterior aspect of the vertebrae. It consists of long fibres running from one end of the ligament to the other and short arched fibres coursing between individual vertebrae. In fact it is inserted into the anterior aspect of the intervertebral disc (3). Thus, facing the anterosuperior and anteroinferior corners of the vertebral bodies lies a potential space (4), where osteophytes are formed in osteoarthrosis.

The posterior longitudinal ligament (5) stetches from the basi-occiput to the sacral canal. Its two edges are festooned as a result of the laterally splayed insertions of its short arched fibres (6) to the posterior aspect of the intervertebral disc. On the contrary, the ligament is not attached to the posterior surface of the vertebrae, leaving a free space traversed by a para-vertebral venous plexus. The concavity of each festoon is related to a pedicle (10).

The sagittal section (fig. 6) reveals the **intervertebral disc** with its annulus fibrosus (8) and its nucleus pulposus (7).

The vertebral arches are joined by segmental ligaments:

each lamina is joined to the next by a thick powerful yellow ligament, the **ligamentum flavum** (11), seen transected (12) in fig. 6. It is inserted inferiorly into the superior border of the underlying lamina and superiorly into the medial aspect of the overlying lamina. Its medial edge fuses with the contralateral ligament in the midline (fig. 8) and completely closes the vertebral canal (11). Anteriorly and laterally it covers the **capsular and the anteromedial ligaments** (14) of the joints between the articular processes. Its anteromedial border therefore skirts the posterior edge of the intervertebral foramen;

the spinous processes are joined by the powerful **interspinous ligament** (15), continuous posteriorly with the **supraspinous ligament** (16), which is attached to the tips of the spinous processes. In the lumbar region the ligament is indistinct as it merges with the crisscrossing insertion fibres of the lumbodorsal muscles;

between the accessory tubercles of the transverse processes lies on either side an **inter-transverse ligament** (17), well developed in the lumbar region.

In fig. 8 the vertebral arch is viewed from in front and the upper vertebra has been detached after sectioning the ligamentum flavum (13). Between the second and third vertebrae the ligament has been totally removed to show the capsule and the anteromedial ligament of the joint between the articular processes (14) and the spinous process.

Taken together these two sets of ligaments constitute an extremely strong link not only between individual vertebrae but also for the vertebral column as a whole.

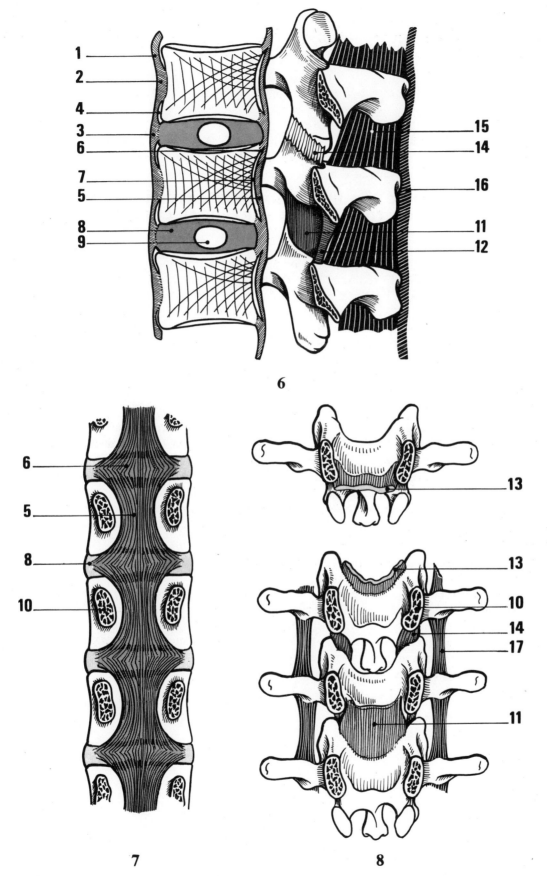

1

7   8

FLEXION AND EXTENSION AND LATERAL FLEXION
OF THE LUMBAR VERTEBRAL COLUMN

During flexion (fig. 9) the body of the upper vertebra tilts and slides gently *anteriorly* in the direction of the arrow F reducing the thickness of the intervertebral disc anteriorly and increasing it posteriorly. The disc therefore becomes wedge-shaped with its base facing posteriorly and the nucleus pulposus is driven *posteriorly* stretching the posterior fibres of the annulus fibrosus. At the same time the inferior articular processes of the upper vertebra slide superiorly and tend to move away from the superior articular processes of the lower vertebra (arrow 1). As a result the ligaments of the joints between these articular processes are maximally stretched as well as all the ligaments of the vertebral arch—the ligamentum flavum, the interspinous ligament (2), the supraspinous ligament and the posterior longitudinal ligament. These stretched ligaments finally limit flexion.

During extension (fig. 10) the body of the upper vertebra tilts and moves posteriorly in the direction of the arrow E. Meanwhile the disc is flattened posteriorly and expanded *anteriorly* and is transformed into a wedge with its base lying anteriorly. The nucleus is pushed anteriorly, stretching the anterior fibres of the annulus and the anterior longitudinal ligament (5) while relaxing the posterior longitudinal ligament. Meanwhile the articular processes of the lower and upper vertebrae become more tightly interlocked and the spinous processes touch one another. Hence extension is limited by the bony structures of the vertebral arch and the tension developed in the anterior longitudinal ligament.

During lateral flexion (fig. 11) the body of the upper vertebra tilts ipsilaterally while the disc becomes wedge-shaped with its base facing contralaterally and the nucleus is slightly displaced contralaterally. The contralateral intertransverse ligament (6) is stretched while the ipsilateral ligament relaxes (7). When view from the back (fig. 12) the articular processes slide relative to each other so that the ipsilateral process of the upper vertebra is raised (8) while the contralateral process is lowered (9). This leads at the same time to relaxation of the contralateral ligamenta flava and of the capsular ligament of the joint between the articular processes and to stretching of these structures ipsilaterally.

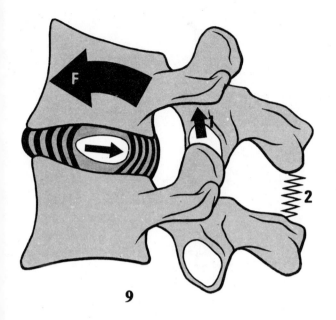

9

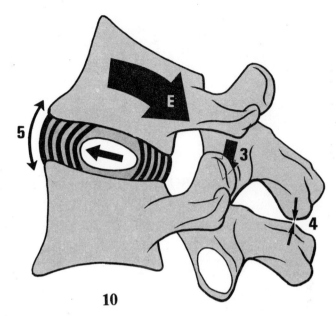

10

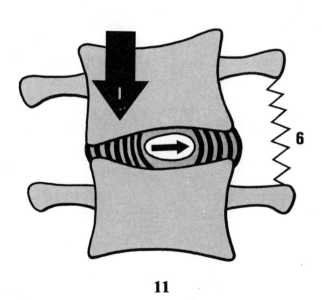

11

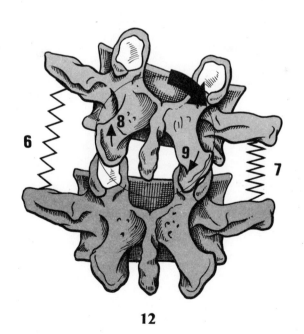

12

ROTATION OF THE LUMBAR VERTEBRAL COLUMN

The articular facets of the superior articular processes of the lumbar vertebrae face posteriorly and medially (fig. 13 and 14: seen from above). They are not flat but concave transversely and straight vertically. Geometrically speaking their profiles correspond to a *cylinder with centre O,* located posteriorly *near the base of the spinous process* (fig. 17). In the case of the upper lumbar vertebrae (fig. 13) the centre of this cylinder lies very near the line joining the posterior borders of the articular processes, whereas for the lower lumbar vertebrae the diameter of this cylinder is much greater so that its centre lies far more posteriorly.

It must be stressed that *the centre of this cylinder does not coincide with the centre of the vertebral plateaus,* so that, when the upper vertebra rotates on the lower vertebra (fig. 15 and 16), this movement of rotation occurs about the former centre and the upper vertebra is found to *slide* over the lower vertebra (fig. 17). The disc (D) is not called into action during axial rotation and this theoretically should allow a greater range of movement. However, the *shearing forces* involved limit the range so that rotation of the lumbar column is minimal both segmentally and globally.

According to Gregersen and D. B. Lucas (see page 119) axial rotation of the lumbar vertebral column would have a total range bilaterally of 10° and so a segmental range of 2° (assuming equal segmental distribution) and a segmental range of 1° for unilateral rotation. It is therefore obvious that the lumbar vertebral column is not built for axial rotation which is sharply limited by the orientation of the articular facets of the vertebrae.

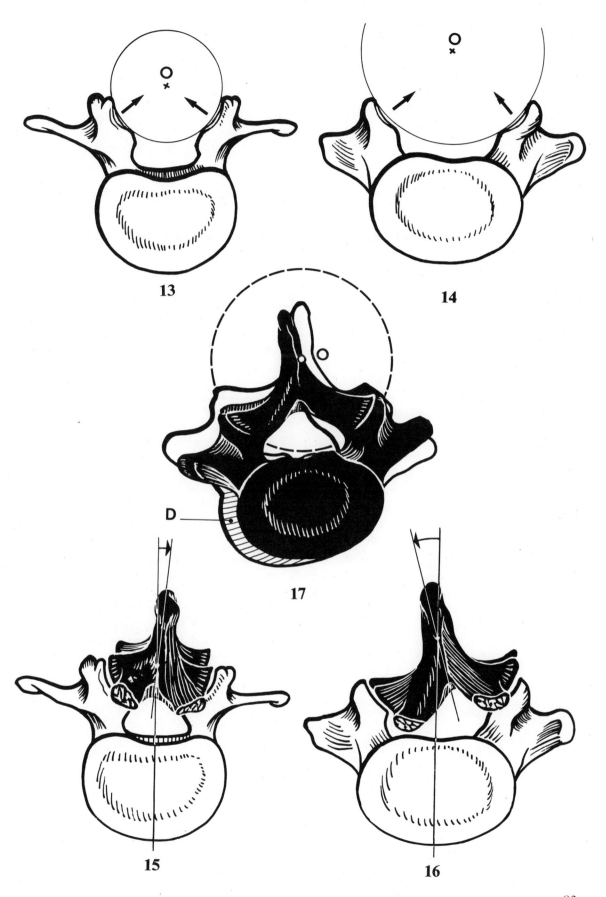

13

14

17

D

15

16

THE LUMBO-SACRAL JOINT AND SPONDYLO-OLISTHESIS

The lumbo-sacral joint is *the weak link in the vertebral column*. In fact (fig. 18), as a result of the inclination of the superior surface of S_1, L_5 tends to slide inferiorly and anteriorly. If the weight P is resolved into its two components—N acting perpendicular to the superior surface of S_1 and G acting parallel—it is obvious that the force G will pull L_5 anteriorly. This is counterbalanced by the powerful anchoring of the vertebral arch of L_5. Viewed from above (fig. 19), the inferior articular processes of L_5 *fit tightly into* the superior articular processes of S_1 and the sliding force G′ tends to bind the vertebral and sacral processes more tightly (the counter-reaction of the sacral processes is expressed as R). These forces act through a point located in the **vertebral isthmus** (fig. 20), which is the part of the vertebral arch lying between the superior and inferior articular processes. If this isthmus is fractured or destroyed (as in fig. 20) the condition is known as *spondylolysis*. As the vertebral arch is no longer retained posteriorly on the superior articular processes of S_1 the body of L_5 slips inferiorly and anteriorly giving rise to *spondylo-olisthesis*. The only structures that still retain L_5 on S_1 and preclude further slippage are, on the one hand, the *lumbosacral disc* with its oblique fibres under tension and, on the other, the *paravertebral muscles* which go into permanent spasm giving rise to the pain of spondylo-olisthesis. The degree of slippage can be measured anteriorly by the degree of overhanging of L_5 relative to the anterior border of S_1.

Special oblique radiographs (fig. 21) show the classical **'small dog'**. Its muzzle is formed by the transverse process, its eye by the pedicle seen end on, its ear by the superior articular process, its paw by the inferior articular process, its tail by the lamina and the contralateral superior articular process, the hind paw by the contralateral inferior articular process and the body by the ipsilateral lamina. It is worth stressing that *the neck represents exactly the vertebral isthmus*. When the isthmus is broken the neck of the dog is cut, establishing the diagnosis of spondylo-olisthesis. Anterior slippage of L_5 must be looked for in oblique views.

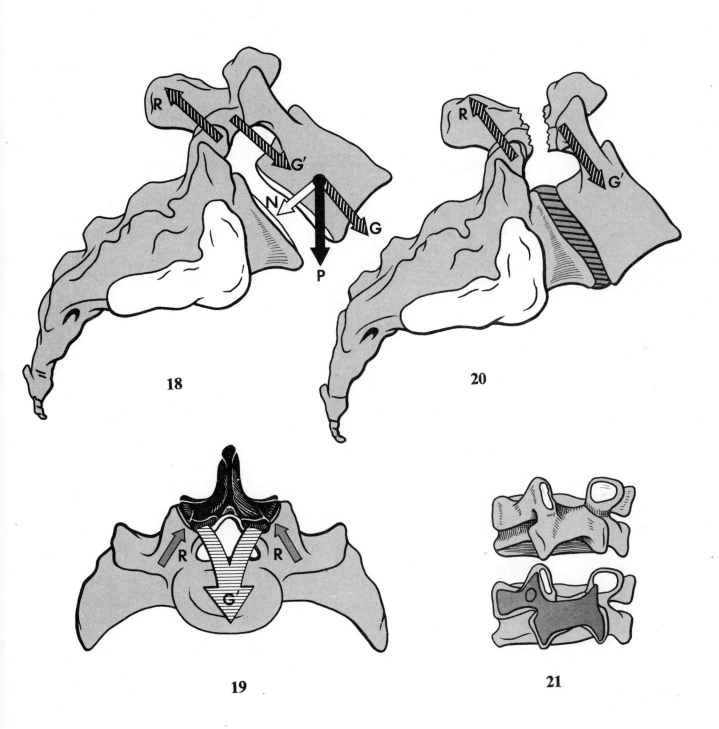

18

20

19

21

ILIOLUMBAR LIGAMENTS AND MOVEMENTS OF THE LUMBOSACRAL JOINT

The last two lumbar vertebrae are joined directly to the iliac bone by the **iliolumbar ligaments** (fig. 22: seen from in front). They have two bands:

the **superior band** (1), attached to the tip of the transverse process of L_4 and running inferiorly, laterally and posteriorly to be inserted into the iliac crest;

the **inferior band** (2), attached to the tip of the transverse process of L_5, and running inferiorly and laterally to be inserted into the iliac crest anteromedially to the superior band. Occasionally two distinct subdivisions can be made out:

a band, strictly iliac (2);

a sacral band (3) which runs more vertically and slightly anteriorly and is attached inferiorly to the anterior surface of the sacro-iliac joint and the most lateral part of the sacral ala.

These iliolumbar ligaments are stretched or relaxed following the movements at the sacro-iliac joint and thus help in limiting these movements.

During lateral flexion (fig. 23: viewed from in front) the iliolumbar ligaments become taut contralaterally and allow only an 8° movement of L_4 relative to the sacrum. The ipsilateral ligaments are relaxed.

During flexion and extension (fig. 24: seen from the side with the iliac bone transparent), the direction of the ligaments is responsible during flexion for the selective stretching of the superior band, which runs an oblique course inferiorly, laterally and posteriorly. Conversely, this band relaxes during extension.

During flexion (F) the inferior band is relaxed as it runs slightly anteriorly and it is stretched during extension (E).

On the whole, movement at the sacro-iliac joint is sharply limited by *the strength of the iliolumbar ligaments*. All things considered, *lateral flexion is more restricted than flexion and extension*.

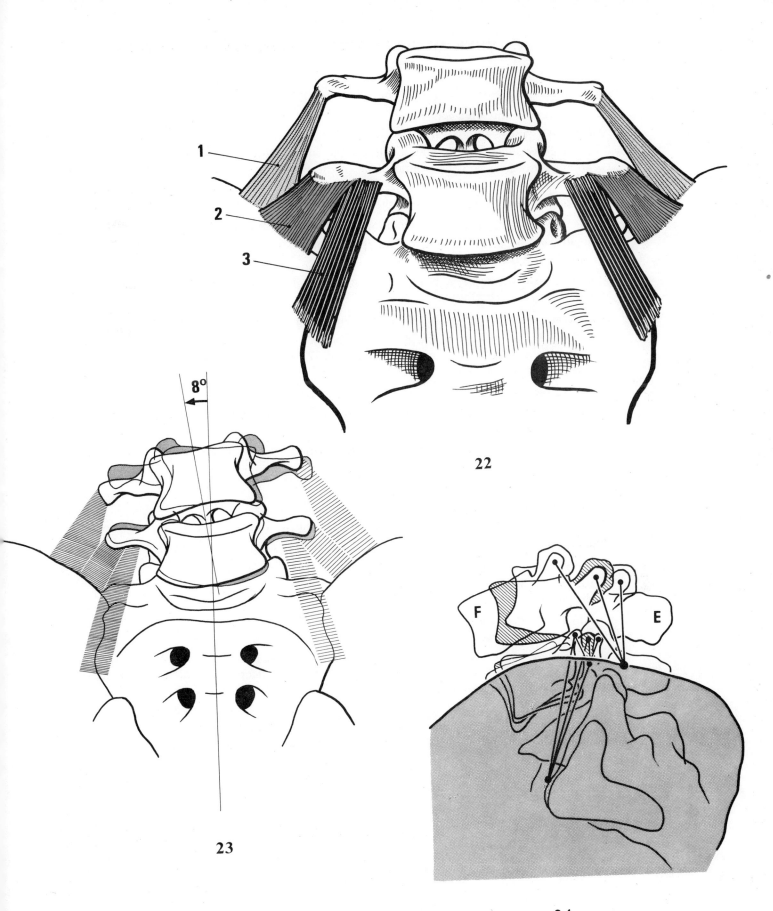

22

23

24

THE TRUNK MUSCLES SEEN IN HORIZONTAL SECTION

A horizontal section passing through L (fig. 25) shows that the muscles fall into three groups.

The posterior muscles consist of:

a *deep plane* which comprises:

the *transversospinalis* (1), which fills up the solid angle between the sagittal plane of the spinous processes and the frontal plane of the transverse processes and is closely moulded on the vertebral laminae;

the longissimus (2), lying lateral to the former;

the iliocostalis (3), a bulky muscle mass lateral to the former;

finally, *the spinalis* (4), attached to the spinous processes and lying posterior to the transversospinalis and the longissimus.

These muscles make up a large fleshy mass that fills up the paravertebral gutters; hence the name paravertebral muscles.

an intermediate plane consisting of the serratus posterior inferior (5);

a superficial plane constituted in the lumbar region by a single muscle, the latissimus dorsi (6), which arises from the very thick lumbar fascia (7), partly attached to the spinous tips. This muscle (6) forms a thick fleshy carpet for the whole posterolateral wall of the lumbar region.

The deep lateral muscles are two in number:

the *quadratus lumborum* (8), attached to the last rib, the transverse processes of the lumbar vertebrae and the iliac crest;

the *psoas* (9), lying within the solid angle formed by the lateral aspects of the vertebral bodies and the transverse processes.

The muscles of the abdominal wall can be subdivided into two groups:

the *medial muscles* (13) lying on either side of the midline;

the *lateral muscles* forming the anterolateral wall of the abdomen.

They are from deep to superficial:

the *transversus abdominis* (10);
the *obliquus internus abdominis* (11);
the *obliquus externus abdominis* (12).

Anteriorly these muscles form an aponeurosis giving rise to the rectus sheath and the linea alba in the following way:

the *aponeurosis of the internal oblique* splits at the lateral border of the rectus abdominis to form two fascial sheets, one superficial (14) and the other deep (15), which enclose the rectus. In the midline these sheets crisscross to form a solid raphe—*the linea alba* (16);

the anterior and posterior sheets of the rectus sheath are reinforced posteriorly by the aponeurosis of the transversus and anteriorly by the aponeurosis of the external oblique. This only applies to the superior part of the abdomen; we shall see later exactly what happens in the inferior part.

The deep lateral muscles and the lateral abdominal muscles bound the *abdominal cavity* into which project the *lumbar vertebral column* (20) and the *large paravertebral vessels* (the aorta and inferior vena cava). The true abdominal cavity (18) is lined by peritoneum, which also lines the posterior aspect of the rectus muscles, the deep aspects of the deep lateral muscles, and the posterior abdominal wall to which are attached the retroperitoneal organs like the *kidneys embedded in retroperitoneal fat* (19). Between the parietal peritoneum and the abdominal wall lies a thin fibrous layer—*the fascia transversalis* (17).

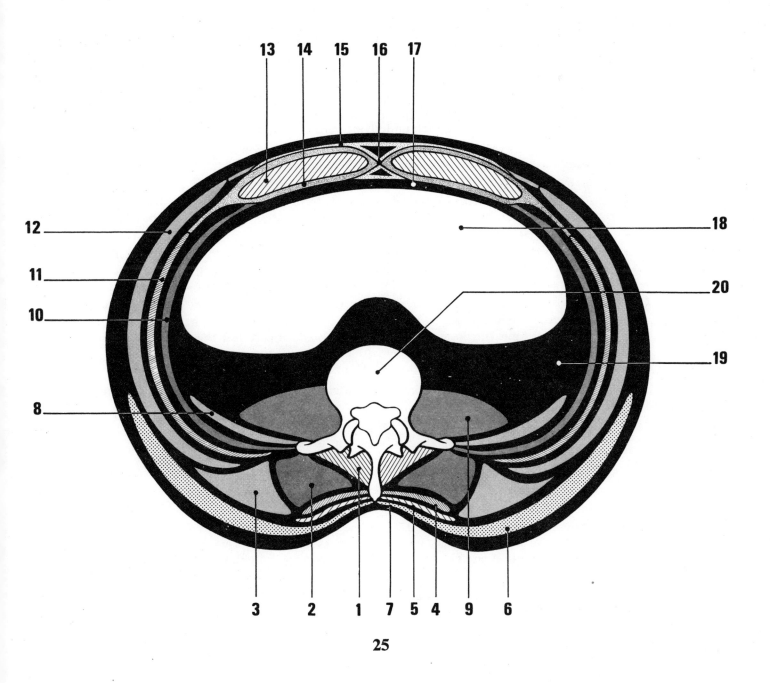

89

POSTERIOR MUSCLES OF THE TRUNK

The posterior muscles of the trunk are arranged in three planes.

The deep plane consists of the spinal muscles which are directly attached to the vertebrae (figs. 26 and 27); hence the name paravertebral. The deeper they lie the shorter is their course.

The transversospinalis (1) is formed of lamellae arranged like tiles on a roof (in the diagram only one lamella is shown). *According to Trolard* the oblique fibres run inferiorly and laterally from the lamina of L_1 to the transverse processes of the underlying four vertebrae. *According to Winckler*, the fibres run from the laminae and spinous processes of the four lumbar vertebrae to the transverse process of each underlying vertebra (see fig. 85, page 239).

The interspinalis muscles (2), which on either side of the midline connect the adjoining spinous processes (the diagram shows only one of these muscles).

The spinalis muscle (3), fusiform in shape, lies on either side of the interspinalis and posterior to the transversospinalis. It arises inferiorly from the upper two lumbar and lower two thoracic spines to be inserted into the spinous processes of the first ten thoracic vertebrae. The deepest fibres run the shortest course.

The longissimus (5), lying lateral to the spinalis, runs in the posterior wall of the thorax to be inserted into the lower 10 ribs (lateral or costal fibres) and into the transverse processes of the lumbar and thoracic vertebrae (medial fibres) [see fig. 29, page 149].

The iliocostalis (6), a thick muscle mass in the shape of a prism, lies posterior and lateral to the above-mentioned muscles. It forms part of the posterior wall of the thorax giving off fibres to be inserted into the posterior aspect of the lower ten ribs near their posterior angles. These fibres are continuous with other fibres that run up to the transverse processes of the lower five cervical vertebrae (see fig. 89, page 241).

In the lower part of the trunk all the muscles are intermingled forming a common muscle mass (6), seen on the right of fig. 27. They are attached to the deep aspect of a thick tendinous sheath which is superficially continuous with the *aponeurosis of the latissimus dorsi* (7).

The intermediate plane (fig. 27) is comprised of only one muscle—the *serratus posterior inferior* (4), lying immediately posterior to the paravertebral muscles and anterior to the latissimus. It arises from transverse processes of the first three lumbar vertebrae and last two thoracic vertebrae and runs an oblique course superiorly and laterally to be inserted into the lower border and lateral aspect of the last three or four ribs.

The superficial plane (fig. 27) is made up of the *latissimus dorsi* (7), which arises from the thick lumbar aponeurosis. Its oblique fibres run superiorly and laterally, cover all the paravertebral muscles and give rise to muscle fibres along an oblique line running inferiorly and medially.

The lumbar aponeurosis as a whole is diamond-shaped with its long axis vertical and its muscle fibres form a broad sheet covering the postero-lateral part of the lower thorax on their way to their humeral insertion (see vol. I).

The action of the posterior muscles is essentially related to extension of the lumbar vertical column (fig. 28). When the sacrum is fixed they powerfully extend the lumbar and thoracic vertebral columns at the lumbosacral joint and at the thoracolumbar joint respectively. In addition they accentuate the lumbar lordosis (fig. 29), as they span *completely or partially* the two ends of the lumbar curvature (fig. 29). It is not correct to say that they straighten the lumbar column. They *pull it posteriorly and increase its curvature*. We shall see later that these muscles are active in expiration.

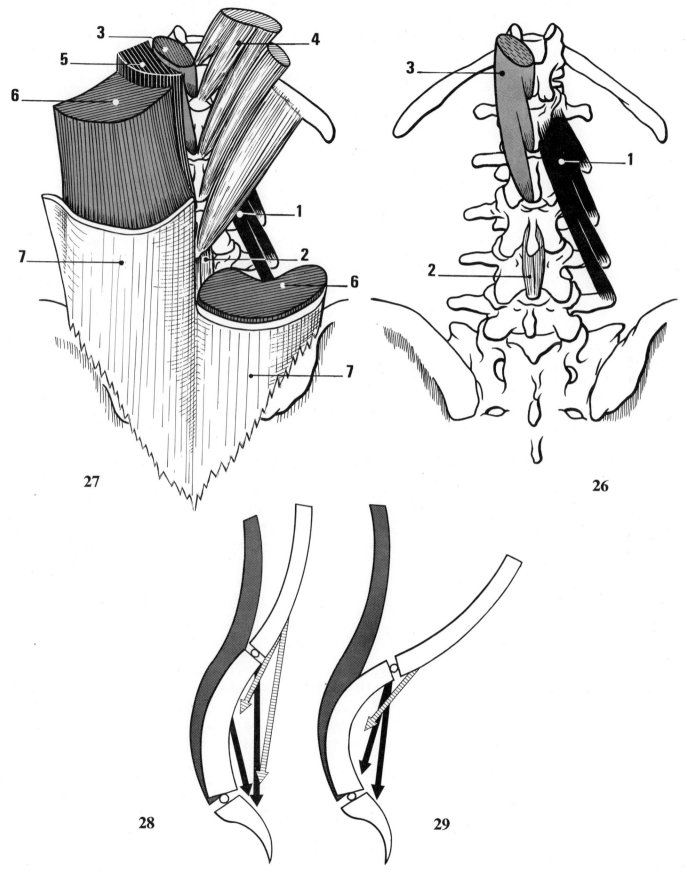

27

26

28

29

ROLE OF THE THIRD LUMBAR AND TWELFTH THORACIC VERTEBRAE

A. Delmas has brought to light the functional significance of certain vertebrae in maintaining the erect position (figs. 30 and 31, according to Delmas). The *wedge shape of L_5*, which acts as a bridge between the more or less horizontal sacrum and the vertical vertebral column, is well-known. On the contrary the *significance of L_3* is just beginning to be appreciated (fig. 30). This vertebra has a better-developed vertebral arch which acts as a *relay station* for, on the one hand, the iliolumbar fibres of the latissimus as they insert into the transverse process of L_3 and, on the other, the ascending fibres of the spinalis whose lowest point of origin is the spinous process of L_3. Hence (fig. 31) L_3 is pulled posteriorly by muscles arising from the sacrum and ilium and can serve as origin for the thoracic muscles. Therefore it is essential in the mechanics of the vertebral column at rest, the more so as it coincides with *the apex of the lumbar curvature* and its *superior and inferior surfaces are parallel and horizontal*. It is the first truly mobile lumbar vertebra as L_4 and L_5, strongly bound to the ilium and sacrum, represent more a static than a dynamic bridge between sacrum and vertebral column.

The twelfth thoracic vertebra, on the other hand, is the point of inflexion between the lumbar and thoracic curvatures. It acts in fact as a swivel and its body is more massive than its vertebral arch, covered posteriorly by the vertebral muscles as they course along without inserting. Delmas considers T_{12} as 'the real swivel of the vertebral axis'.

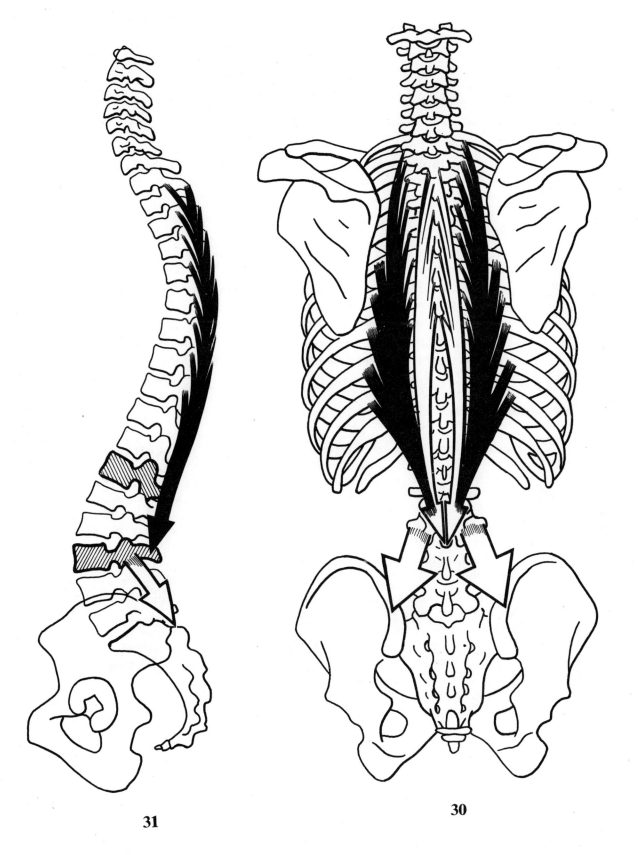

31

30

THE LATERAL MUSCLES OF THE TRUNK

The lateral muscles are *two in number*: the quadratus lumborum and the psoas.

The quadratus lumborum (fig. 32, viewed from in front) forms, as the name implies, a quadrilateral sheet of muscle running between the last rib, the iliac crest and the vertebral column and having a free superficial border. It is made up of three sets of fibres (right side of figure):

fibres running directly between the last rib and the iliac crest (white arrows);

fibres running between the last rib and the transverse processes of the five lumbar vertebrae (hatched arrows running transversely);

fibres running between the transverse processes of the first four lumbar vertebrae to the iliac crest (stippled grey arrows). These fibres are continuous with those of the transversospinalis (black arrow) as they emerge between the transverse processes.

These three sets of fibres are also arranged in three planes—the posterior plane consisting of the iliocostal fibres, the intermediate plane of the iliovertebral fibres and the anterior plane of the costovertebral fibres (1).

When one quadratus contracts it *flexes* the trunk ipsilaterally (fig. 33). It is powerfully helped in this movement by the internal oblique (stippled grey arrow pointing inferolaterally) and the external oblique (hatched arrow pointing inferomedially).

The **psoas** lies anterior to the quadratus (fig. 34) and its fusiform muscle belly takes origin as two separate muscle sheets: a posterior sheet attached to the transverse processes of the lumbar vertebrae, and an anterior sheet attached to the bodies of T_{12} and lumbar vertebrae. These latter fibres are attached to the inferior and superior borders of two contiguous vertebrae and to the lateral border of the intervertebral disc. Tendinous arches bridge over these separate muscle attachments. The fusiform body of the muscle, flattened anteroposteriorly, runs an oblique course inferiorly and laterally, follows the pelvic brim, is reflected on the anterior edge of the hip bone over the iliopubic eminence, and, along with the iliacus, gains insertion into the tip of the lesser trochanter.

If the femur is fixed and the hip is stabilised by contraction of other periarticular muscles, the psoas has a *very powerful effect on the lumbar vertebral column* (fig. 35), leading to *lateral flexion ipsilaterally and rotation contralaterally*. Furthermore (fig. 36), as it is attached to the summit of the lumbar curvature, it also brings about *flexion* of the vertebral column relative to the pelvis and *accentuates* the lumbar lordosis, as clearly seen in a subject lying supine with the lower limbs at rest (see fig. 62, page 113).

On the whole, the lateral muscles flex the trunk ipsilaterally but, whereas the quadratus has no effect on the lumbar lordosis, the psoas accentuates it and causes the column to rotate contralaterally.

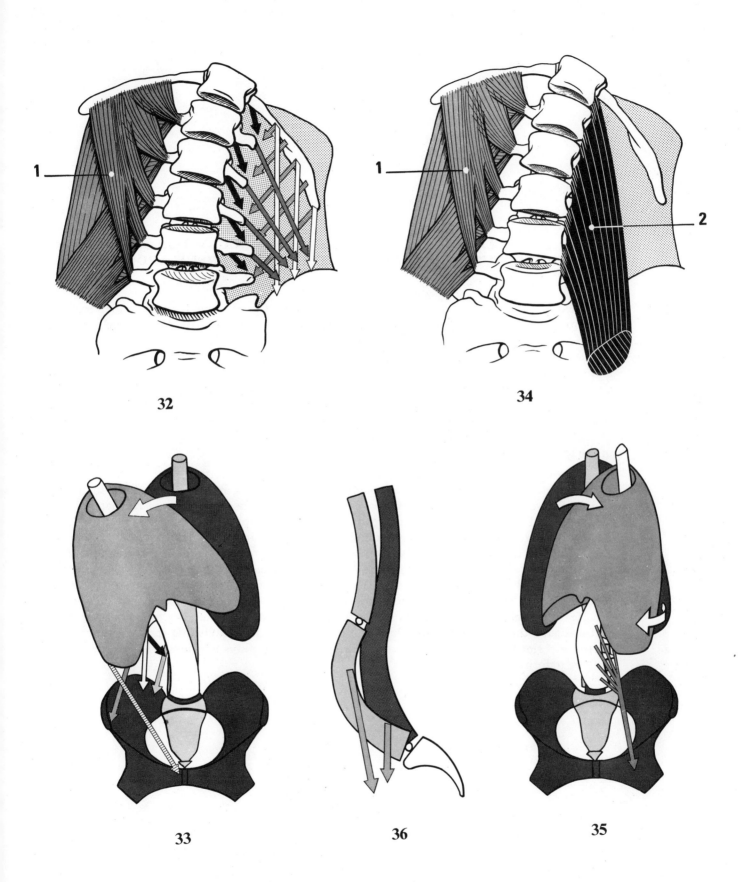

32

34

33

36

35

THE MUSCLES OF THE ABDOMINAL WALL:
THE RECTUS ABDOMINIS AND THE TRANSVERSUS ABDOMINIS

The two rectus muscles (fig. 37 seen from in front, fig. 38 seen from the side) make up two muscle sheets lying *in the anterior abdominal wall* on either side of the midline. They are inserted as a thick wide band into the anterior arches and costal cartilages of the fifth, sixth and seventh ribs and into the xiphoid process. Below its insertion the muscle narrows gradually and is interrupted by aponeurotic intersections (two at the level of the umbilicus, one above and one below). The infraumbilical portion of the muscle is clearly narrower and it tapers down into a powerful tendon attached to the pubic crest, the pubic symphysis and by lateral expansions to the opposite side. The rectus muscles are separated across the midline by a greater distance above than below. They are contained within an aponeurotic sheath formed by the aponeuroses of the abdominal muscles.

The **transversus abdominis** (fig. 39, seen from in front; fig. 40 seen from the side) forms the deepest layer of the lateral abdominal muscles. It is attached posteriorly to the tips of the transverse processes of the lumbar vertebrae and its horizontal fibres run laterally and anteriorly and surround the internal organs. It breaks up into an aponeurosis along the lateral border of the rectus and crosses the midline to merge with its fellow on the opposite side. For the most part the aponeurosis lies deep to the rectus contributing to the formation of the *posterior wall of the rectus sheath*. However, *below the umbilicus* the aponeurosis runs superficial to the rectus which perforates the transversus so as to gain access to its deep surface. From this level down, the aponeurosis contributes to the *anterior wall of the rectus sheath*. In the diagram it is clear that only the middle fibres run horizontally; the oblique superior fibres run superiorly and medially, the oblique inferior fibres run inferiorly and medially while the lowest fibres end on the superior border of the pubic symphysis and of the pubis and join those of the internal oblique to form the conjoint tendon.

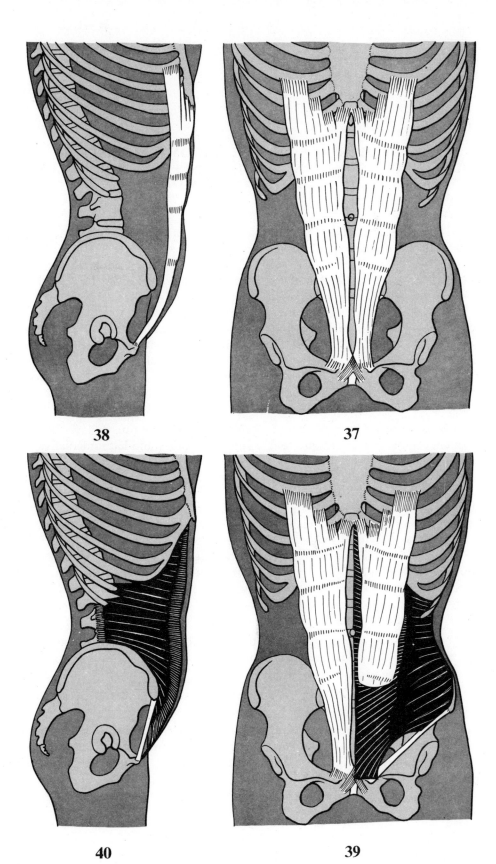

38

37

40

39

THE MUSCLES OF THE ABDOMINAL WALL:
THE OBLIQUUS INTERNUS ABDOMINIS AND THE OBLIQUUS EXTERNUS ABDOMINIS

The **internal oblique** (figs. 41 and 42) makes up the intermediate layer of the muscles of the abdominal wall. Its fibres in general run an oblique course superoinferiorly and lateromedially and are attached to the iliac crest. The muscle fibres form a sheet covering the lateral wall of the abdomen and some are attached directly to the eleventh and twelfth ribs and others indirectly via an *aponeurosis* formed along a line running from the tip of the eleventh rib and vertically along the lateral edge of the rectus. These aponeurotic fibres are attached to the tenth costal cartilage and xiphoid process and contribute to the *anterior wall of the rectus sheath*. They also cross the midline to merge with similar fibres from the opposite side and form the *linea alba*. The lowest fibres of the muscle, attached directly to the inguinal ligament, are at first horizontal and then oblique inferiorly and medially and they form the *conjoint tendon* along with the transversus before gaining attachment to the superior border of the pubic symphysis and the pubic crest. The conjoint tendon thus forms part of the wall of the deep inguinal ring.

The **external oblique** (figs. 43 and 44) forms the superficial muscle layer of the abdominal wall. Its fibres in general run an oblique course superoinferiorly and lateromedially. It arises from the lower ribs by fleshy fibres, which interdigitate with those of the serratus anterior. These fibres, partially overlapping one another in an inferosuperior direction form part of the lateral abdominal wall and give rise to an *aponeurosis* along a line of transition, which is at first vertical, then parallel to the lateral border of the rectus and, finally, oblique inferiorly and posteriorly. This aponeurosis contributes to the *anterior wall of the rectus sheath* and meets with similar fibres from the other side to help form the *linea alba*. The fibres arising from the ninth rib are attached to the pubis and send aponeurotic expansions towards the origins of the ipsilateral and contra-lateral adductors of the thigh. The fibres arising from the tenth rib join the inguinal ligament to form the *superficial inguinal ring*, which is a triangular opening with its apex facing superolaterally and its inferomedial base constituted by the pubis and the pubic tubercle which receives the attachment of the inguinal ligament.

From this description of the muscles of the abdominal wall; which constitute the anterior group of the motor muscles of the vertebral column, the following should be singled out:

the rectus muscles, lying anteriorly in the anterior abdominal wall, form two muscle bands which are *far removed from the vertebral column*, and bridge the gap between the base of the thoracic cavity and the anterior part of the bony pelvis.

the lateral muscles are arranged in three layers with their muscle fibres running in different directions: in the deep layer (transversus) the fibres are transverse; in the intermediate layer (internal oblique) they are oblique superiorly and medially; in the superficial layer (external oblique) they are oblique inferiorly and medially (see fig. 31, page 151).

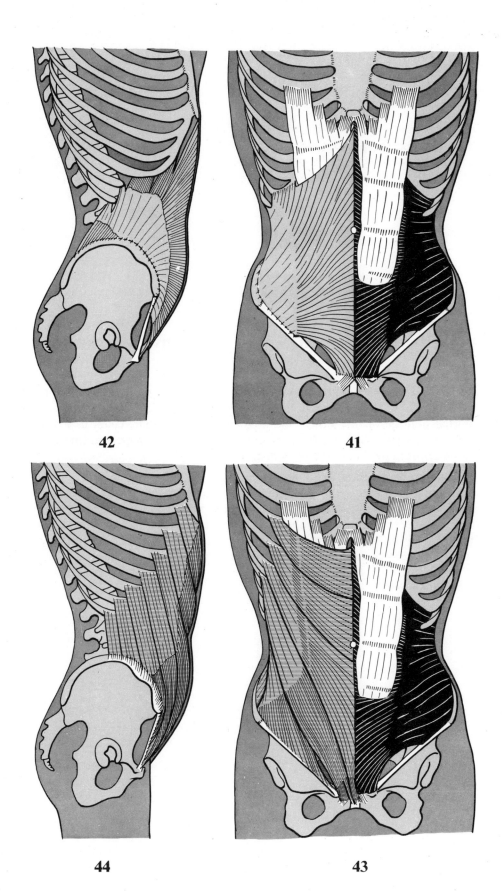

42

41

44

43

MUSCLES OF THE ABDOMINAL WALL: THE CURVE OF THE WAIST

The fibres of the lateral muscles and their aponeuroses form a *real girdle* around the abdomen (fig. 45). In fact, the fibres of the external oblique on one side are directly continuous with the fibres of the internal oblique on the other side and vice versa so that, taken as a whole, the oblique muscles form a carpet which is not rectangular but diamond-shaped and lies on a *slant*. This slant in fact determines the hollow of the waist.

This can be easily demonstrated on a model (fig. 46). If strings or elastic bands (A) are drawn between two circles parallel to the axis joining the centres of the two circles, a cylindrical surface is obtained. If the upper circle is rotated relative to the lower circle (B) the strings remain taut but run obliquely and the envelope of the surface described is known as a *hyperboloid of revolution*. Its surface is hollowed in the form of a hyperbolic curve. This explains why the waist is hollow, the more so as the oblique fibres are under stronger tension and the subcutaneous fat is thinner. Therefore to restore the hollow of the waist one must build up the tone of the oblique muscles of the abdomen.

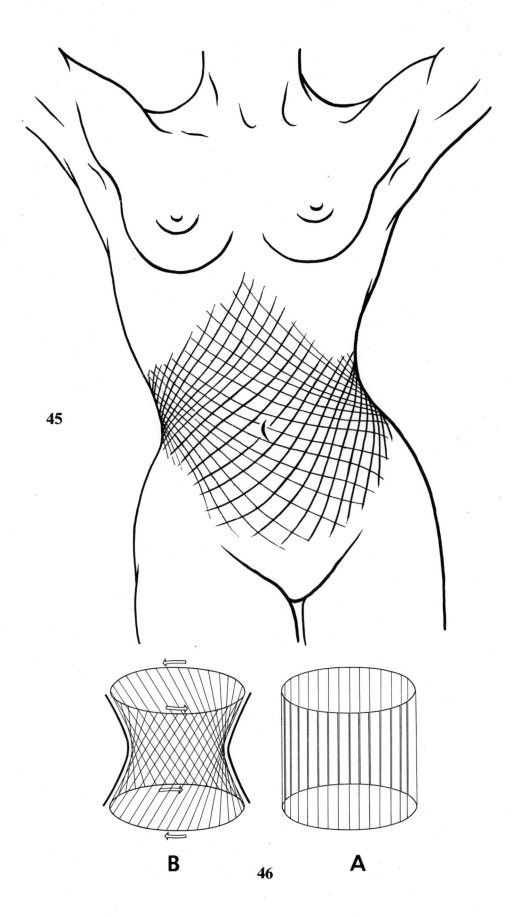

45

B   46   A

MUSCLES OF THE ABDOMINAL WALL: ROTATION OF THE TRUNK

Rotation of the vertebral column is achieved by the *paravertebral muscles* and the *lateral muscles of the abdomen*. Unilateral contraction of the paravertebral muscles causes only weak rotation, but the deepest muscle layer—the transversospinalis (T.S.)—is more effective. When its origin from the underlying transverse process is fixed, it pulls the spinous process of the overlying vertebra laterally. Therefore it causes rotation on the opposite side.

During rotation of the trunk, the main muscles involved are the *oblique muscles* (fig. 48). Their mechanical efficiency is enhanced by their spiral course around the waist and by their attachments to the thoracic cage away from the vertebral column, so that both the lumbar and the lower thoracic vertebral columns are mobilised. *To rotate the trunk to the left* (fig. 48) both the *right* external oblique and the *left* internal oblique are needed. It is worth noting that these muscles are wrapped round the waist in the same direction (fig. 49) and that their muscle fibres and aponeuroses are continuous in the same direction. They are therefore *synergistic* for this movement.

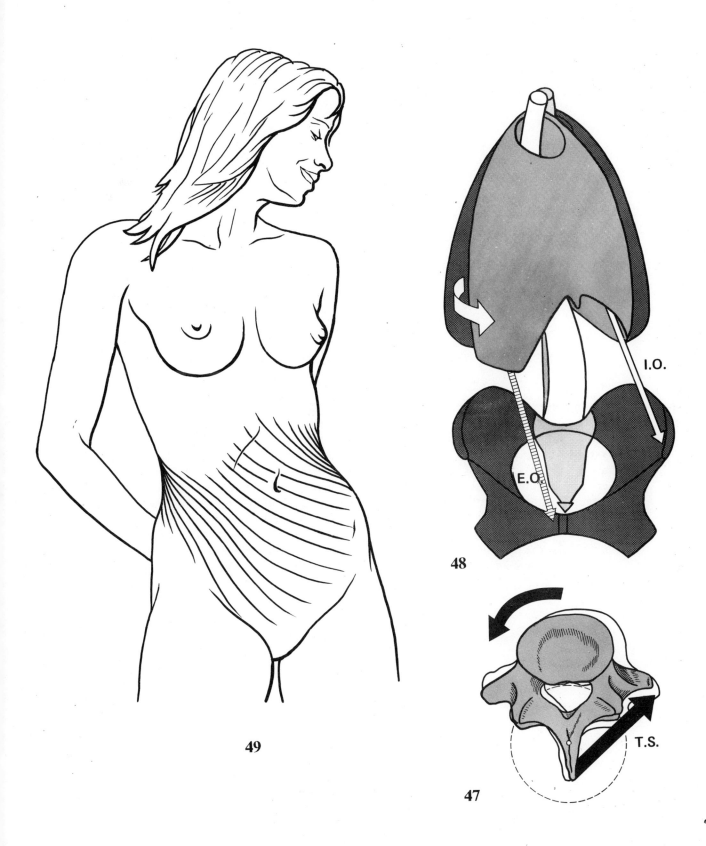

I.O.

E.O.

48

T.S.

47

49

103

MUSCLES OF THE ABDOMINAL WALL: FLEXION OF THE TRUNK

The muscles of the abdominal wall are *powerful flexors of the trunk* (fig. 50). Lying anterior to the axis of the vertebral column they pull the whole column forward at the lumbosacral and thoracolumbar joints. Their power lies in the fact that they operate by means of **a lever system**: the *inferior arm of the lever* corresponds to the distance between the sacral promontory and the pubic symphysis; *the superior arm of the lever* to the distance between the thoracic vertebral column and the xiphoid process (shown in the diagram as a bracket resting on the vertebral column). The rectus (R), which links the xiphoid and the pubic symphysis directly is a powerful flexor and is helped by the internal (I.O.) and the external (E.O.) obliques which link the lower border of the thoracic cage and the bony pelvis. Whereas the rectus acts as a *direct brace,* the internal oblique acts as an *oblique brace inferiorly and posteriorly* and the external oblique as a *brace inferiorly and anteriorly.* These also act as *stays* because of their obliquity.

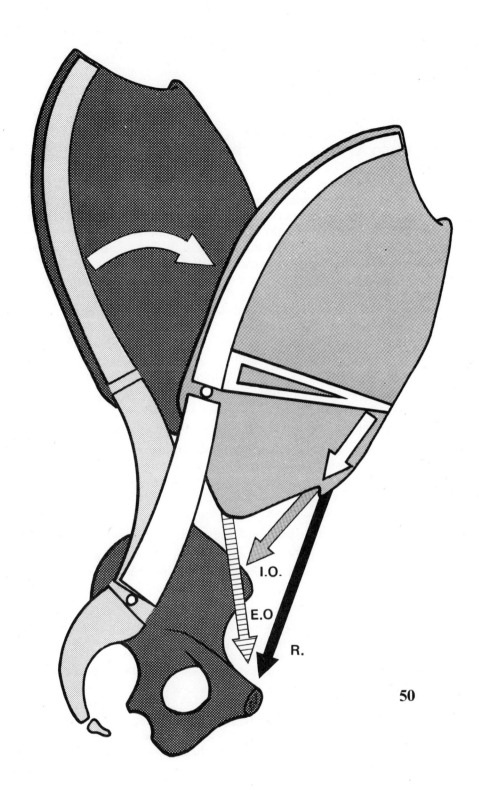

I.O.

E.O

R.

50

MUSCLES OF THE ABDOMINAL WALL:
THE FLATTENING OF THE LUMBAR CURVATURE

The variable lumbar curvature depends not only on the tone of the abdominal and paravertebral muscles but also on some lower limb muscles attached to the bony pelvis. In the *asthenic subject* (fig. 51B) the muscle relaxation accentuates all three spinal curvatures, i.e., lumbar, thoracic and cervical. Also the pelvis *tilts anteriorly* and the interspinous line, joining the anterosuperior iliac spine to the posterosuperior iliac spine, becomes oblique inferiorly and anteriorly. The psoas (P), which flexes the vertebral column relative to the pelvis and accentuates the lumbar curvature, becomes hypertonic and further aggravates the abnormal posture. This asthenic stance is often seen in people without energy or will-power. Similar changes in the vertebral column also obtain in late pregnancy when the resting position of the vertebral column and pelvis is considerably disturbed by stretching of the abdominal wall and the forward displacement of the centre of gravity of the body as a result of the enlarging foetus.

Flattening of spinal curvatures (fig. 51A) is initiated at the level of the pelvis. The forward tilt of the pelvis is counterbalanced by the *extensor muscles of the hip*. As the *hamstrings* (H) and *gluteus maximus* (GM) contract they tilt the pelvis posteriorly and restore the interspinous line to the horizontal plane. The sacrum also becomes vertical and this reduces the lumbar curvature.

The crucial muscles in this process are the abdominal muscles, particularly the *rectus muscles* (R), which span the two ends of the lumbar curvature and act, as already shown, like a lever. Therefore contraction of the rectus and gluteus muscles is enough to flatten the lumbar curvature. From this point onwards, contraction of the paravertebral muscles (S), i.e., acting to extend the column, can pull back the upper lumbar vertebrae.

The thoracic curvature is flattened by the action of the posterior muscles of the trunk.

Similarly the cervical curvature is flattened by the action of the paravertebral muscles, as will be discussed later. On the whole, as the curvatures flatten, the vertebral column grows longer by 1–3 cm (corresponding to a slight increase in the Delmas index).

This is the accepted theory but recent quantitative studies (Klausen, 1965) indicate that the column taken as a whole behaves like the *shaft of a crane* overhanging anteriorly. Simultaneous electromyographic recordings of the posterior muscles of the trunk and of the abdominal muscles (Asmussen and Klausen 1962) show that in 80 per cent of cases the standing posture, reflexly maintained, depends only on tonic activity of the posterior muscles. If one loads the upper part of the vertebral column by placing a weight on the head or carrying weights in the hands hanging freely along the trunk, the anterior overhanging of the column is slightly accentuated leading to an increase in the cervical curvature and a decrease in the lumbar curvature. At the same time the paravertebral muscles increase their tone to counteract this effect. Therefore, the abdominal muscles do not actively support the vertebral column at rest but they are recruited when the lumbar curvature is consciously flattened, i.e., as when standing to attention or when heavy weights are carried with the trunk flexed.

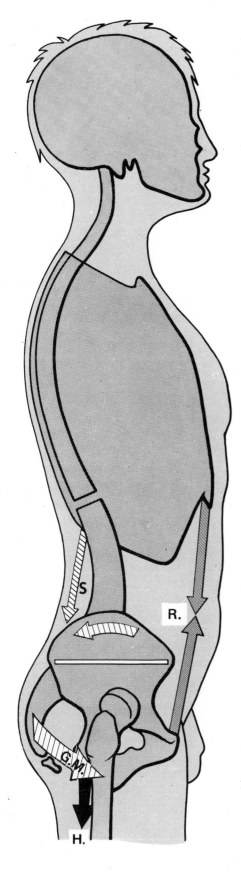

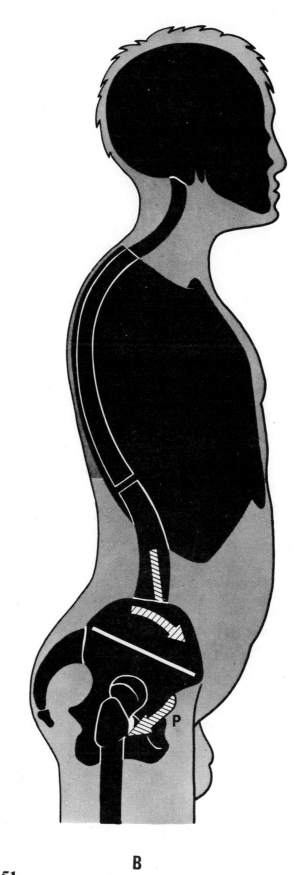

A
      51   B

THE TRUNK AS AN INFLATABLE STRUCTURE

During forward flexion, if only the paravertebral muscles are active, the stresses on the lumbosacral disc are *considerable*. In fact, the weight of the upper part of the trunk and the head acts through the partial centre of gravity (P) lying just posterior to T_{10}. This weight (P_1) is applied at the tip of the long arm of a lever with its fulcrum at the level of the nucleus pulposus of L_5–S_1. To counterbalance this force the paravertebral muscles (S_1), acting on the short arm of the lever 7 to 8 times shorter than the long arm, must develop a force 7 to 8 times greater than P_1. This force will vary according to the degree of flexion of the trunk as it alters the length of the long arm on which P_1 is acting. Anyway the force acting on the lumbosacral disc is equal to $S_1 + P_1$. It increases progressively with the degree of flexion or with the carrying of weights in the hands.

To lift a 10 kg weight, with flexed knees and the trunk held vertically, the force S_1 exerted by the paravertebral muscles amounts to 141 kg. Lifting the same weight with extended knees and trunk flexed forward, requires a force of 256 kg. If again this same weight is carried with the arms outstretched anteriorly, S_1 equals 363 kg. At this time it is believed that the force acting on the lumbosacral disc ranges from 282 to 726 kg or even up to 1200 kg, the latter value clearly exceeding the force required to smash the intervertebral discs (800 kg in the young, 450 kg in the aged).

This apparent contradiction can be explained in two ways. Firstly, the full impact of the force is not borne by the nucleus of the disc. Nachemson has shown that, when a force is applied to a disc, it is distributed as follows: 75 per cent on the nucleus, 25 per cent on the annulus.

Secondly, the *trunk as a whole intervenes* to relieve the pressure applied to the lumbosacral and lower lumbar discs (fig. 52B). It is worthy of note that, when one lifts a weight, one instinctively performs a *Valsalva manoeuvre* which consists of closing the glottis and all the abdominal orifices. This turns the thoraco-abdominal cavity into a closed cavity stabilised by the contraction of the expiratory muscles, in particular the *abdominal muscles*. Thus the pressure rises considerably within the cavity and transforms it into a *rigid beam* lying anterior to the vertebral column and transmitting the forces exerted on the bony pelvis and the perineum. The recruitment of this **inflatable structure** markedly reduces the axial compression forces acting on the disc, i.e., by 50 per cent for disc T_2–L_1 and 30 per cent for disc L_5–S_1. For the same reason, the force exerted by the paravertebral muscles is decreased by 55 per cent. This mechanism is therefore very useful in protecting the vertebral column but it is active for a very short time. It calls for *complete apnoea* which leads to important cardiovascular disturbances, i.e., *cerebral venous hypertension, decrease in venous return, decrease in pulmonary capillary blood flow* and *increase in pulmonary vascular resistance*. It also presupposes that the muscles of the abdominal girdle are intact and that the glottis and abdominal orifices can be closed. Finally the pressure rise in the thoraco-abdominal cavity shunts blood into the *vertebral venous plexus* and as a result *raises the pressure of the cerebrospinal fluid*. Such a situation cannot be maintained indefinitely and the *lifting of heavy weights can only be brief and intense*. The practical lesson to be drawn is that to reduce the pressure acting on the intervertebral discs, it is better to lift weights with the trunk vertical rather than flexed forward. This is the advice that must be given to people suffering from slipped discs.

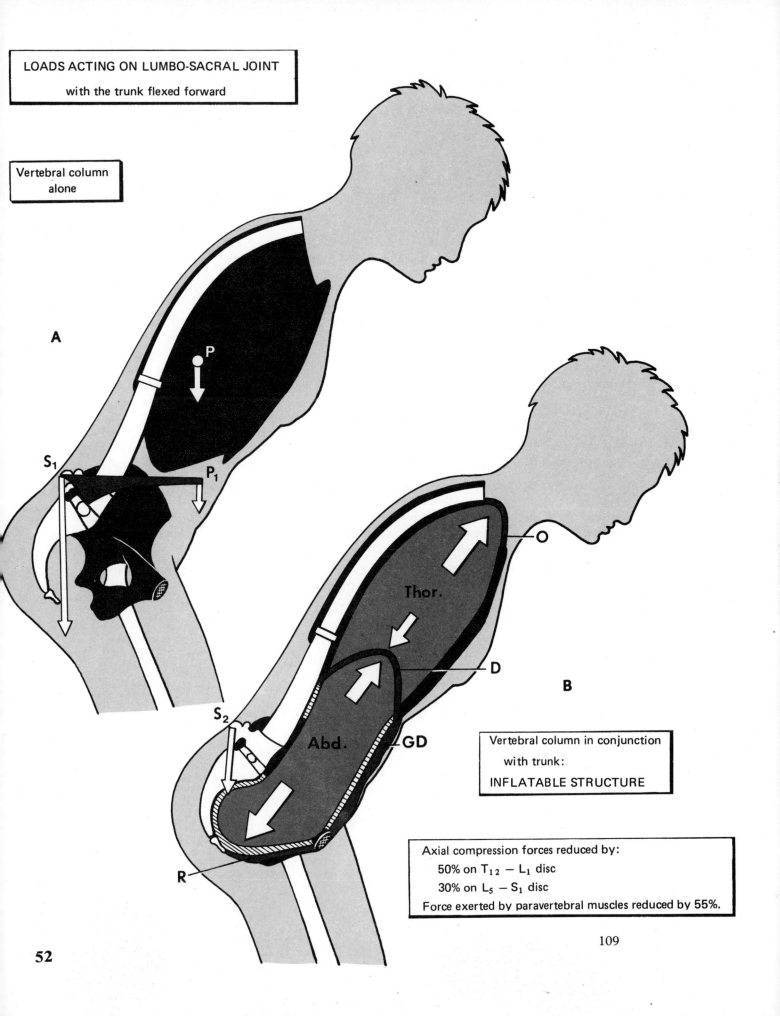

LOADS ACTING ON LUMBO-SACRAL JOINT

with the trunk flexed forward

Vertebral column alone

A

P

S_1

P_1

S_2

Thor.

O

D

B

Abd.

GD

R

Vertebral column in conjunction with trunk:

INFLATABLE STRUCTURE

Axial compression forces reduced by:

50% on $T_{12} - L_1$ disc

30% on $L_5 - S_1$ disc

Force exerted by paravertebral muscles reduced by 55%.

THE VERTEBRAL COLUMN WHILE STANDING AT REST

When the body is supported **symmetrically** on both lower limbs the lumbar vertebral column seen from the side (fig. 53) shows a curve convex anteriorly, i.e., the lumbar lordosis. From the back (fig. 54) it is straight and when the body is **asymmetrically** supported on one lower limb (fig. 55) the column shows a curve concave towards the supporting limb as a result of tilting of the pelvis so that the supporting hip lies higher than the resting hip. To compensate for this lumbar lateral flexion the thoracic column is flexed in the opposite direction, i.e., towards the resting limb. Finally the cervical column shows a curve similar to the lumbar one.

Electromyographic studies by Brügger show that during **flexion of the trunk** (fig. 56) the paravertebral muscles are the first to contract powerfully, then the glutei, and finally the hamstrings and the soleus muscles. At the end of flexion the vertebral column is stabilised only by the *passive action of vertebral ligaments* (L) fixed to the bony pelvis, which is tilted forward by the hamstrings (H).

When the trunk is righted (fig. 57) the order of muscle recruitment is the converse: first the hamstrings, then the glutei and finally the lumbar and thoracic muscles (S).

When one stands up straight (fig. 58), there is a slightly forward bias which is counter-balanced by tonic contraction of the posterior muscles of the trunk, the gastrocnemius and soleus (the triceps surae T), the hamstrings (H) and the spinal muscles (S) with the abdominal muscles in a state of relaxation (Asmussen).

110

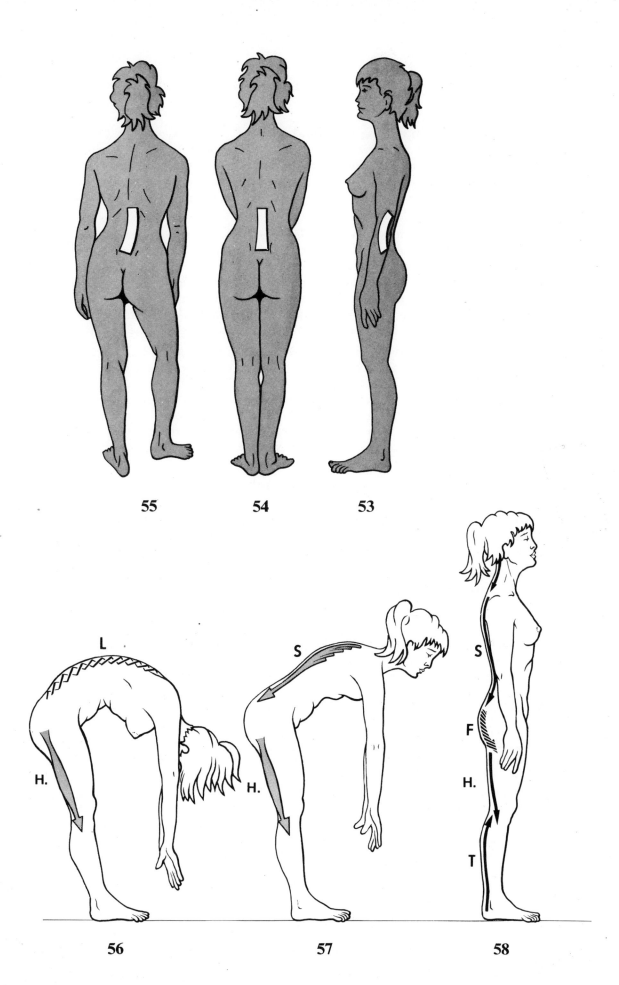

55   54   53

56   57   58

In the sitting position relying on ischial support, as when *typing* (fig. 59) without resting on the back of the chair, the weight of the trunk is borne only by the ischial bones and the pelvis is *in a state of unstable equilibrium* with a tendency to tilt forward leading to an accentuation of three vertebral curvatures. As a result, the scapular muscles, especially the *trapezius*, are called into action to stabilise the vertebral column. In the long run this position becomes painful and the condition is known as the typist's syndrome or the trapezius syndrome.

In the sitting position, relying on ischio-femoral support (fig. 60), the flexed trunk is supported by the ischial tuberosities and the posterior aspects of the thighs, though on occasions the trunk may be supported by the arms resting on the knees. The pelvis is tilted forward and the accentuation of the thoracic curvature leads to a flattening of the lumbar curvature. If the arms act as stays, the trunk is stable with minimal muscular support and one can even fall asleep. *As it rests the paravertebral muscles*, it is often assumed by patients with spondyloolisthesis. This *decreases the shearing forces* on the lumbosacral disc and relaxes the posterior muscles.

In the sitting position relying on ischio-sacral support (fig. 61), the trunk is pulled back as a whole to rest on the back of the chair and is supported by the ischial tuberosities, the posterior surface of the sacrum and the coccyx. The pelvis is tilted backwards, the lumbar curvature is flattened, the thoracic curvature is increased and the head may lie forward on the thorax leading to inversion of the cervical curvature. This is a position where sleep is possible but breathing is hampered by neck flexion and the weight of the head resting on the sternum. This position reduces slippage of L_5 and relaxes the posterior muscles and relieves the pain of spondyloolisthesis.

The supine position with extended limbs (fig. 62) is the most commonly adopted posture for resting. The psoas is stretched and accentuates the lumbar curvature hollowing the loin.

In the supine position with flexed lower limbs (fig. 63) relaxation of the psoas causes a backward tilt of the pelvis and a flattening of the lumbar curvature. The loin rests on the supporting surface and relaxes even better the spinal and abdominal muscles.

In the so-called position of relaxation (fig. 64), achieved with the help of cushions or specially designed chairs, the thoracic curvature is accentuated with flattening of the lumbar and cervical curvatures. If the knees are supported the hips are flexed and the psoas and hamstrings are relaxed.

When one lies on the side (fig. 65), the vertebral column becomes curved. The line perpendicular to the tangent at the apex of the lumbar convexity, the line joining the two posterosuperior iliac spines (surface marked by the sacral dimples) and the interscapular line converge at a point above the subject. The thoracic vertebral column becomes convex superiorly. This position cannot relax all the muscles and causes respiratory difficulties during anaesthesia.

The prone position is bedevilled by the adverse consequences of an exaggerated lumbar curvature and by *respiratory difficulties*. The latter result from the pressure of the supporting surface on the thorax and abdomen, pushing back the viscera on to the diaphragm and reducing its excursion, and from obstruction of the lower trachea, i.e., the carina, by secretions or an inhaled foreign body. Many people adopt this position to go to sleep and later change. In general a single position is never kept for a long time during sleep and this is to allow the *successive relaxation of muscular groups* and a *constant change of the pressure areas*. It is well known that if the same areas are under pressure for over three hours ischaemic pressure sores will develop.

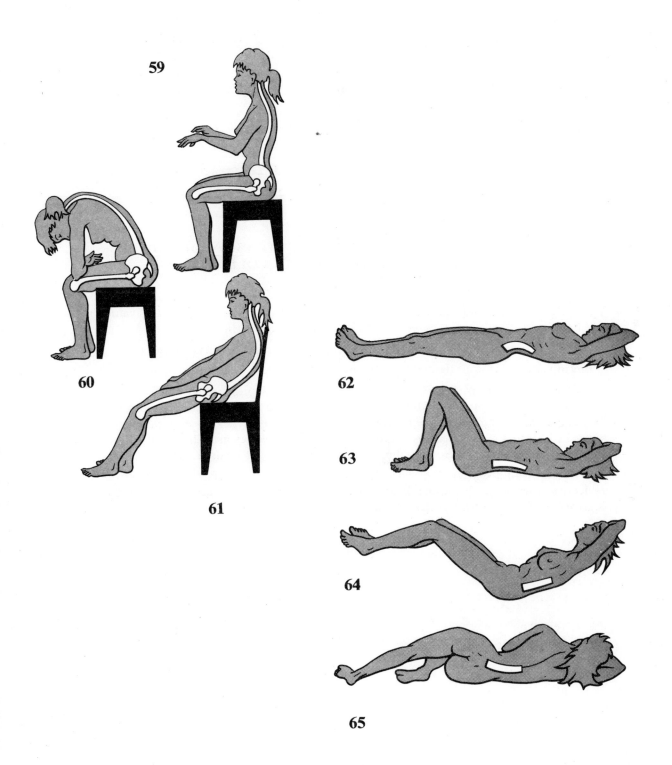

59

60

61

62

63

64

65

113

RANGE OF FLEXION AND EXTENSION OF THE
LUMBAR VERTEBRAL COLUMN

The range of these movements *varies with the subject and with age*. All the values presented are therefore particular cases or averages. For example (fig. 66):

extension associated with accentuation of the lumbar curvature has a range of 30°;

flexion associated with flattening of the lumbar curvature, has a range of 40°.

David and Allbrook (fig. 67A) have established the individual ranges of flexion and extension at each segment (right side). The total cumulative range of flexion and extension (left side) is 83°, i.e., close to the value mentioned above. The range of flexion and extension is maximal between L_4 and L_5, and decreases progressively at higher levels. Therefore the lower lumbar column is more active in flexion and extension than the upper column.

As one would expect, the *range of flexion varies with age* (fig. 67B, according to Tanz). It decreases with age, being maximal between two and thirteen years of age. Again movement is greater in the lower part of the lumbar column, especially at level L_4–L_5.

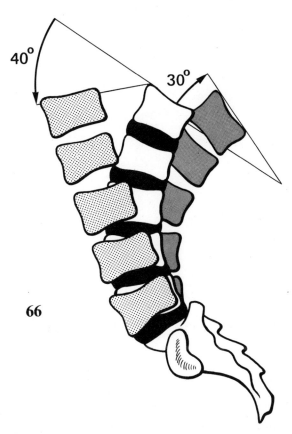

40°   30°

66

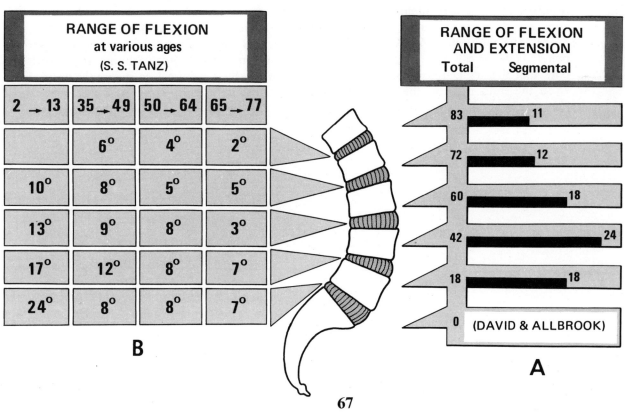

RANGE OF FLEXION at various ages (S. S. TANZ)			
2 → 13	35 → 49	50 → 64	65 → 77
	6°	4°	2°
10°	8°	5°	5°
13°	9°	8°	3°
17°	12°	8°	7°
24°	8°	8°	7°

B

RANGE OF FLEXION AND EXTENSION	
Total	Segmental
83	11
72	12
60	18
42	24
18	18
0	(DAVID & ALLBROOK)

A

67

RANGE OF LATERAL FLEXION OF THE LUMBAR VERTEBRAL COLUMN

As with flexion and extension, the range of **lateral flexion** varies with the individual and with age. On the average the range falls between 20 and 30°.

According to Tanz (fig. 69), it decreases with age, being maximal between two and thirteen years of age, when it amounts to 62° on either side of the midline. Between 35 and 49 years it falls to 30°, between 50 and 64 years to 29°, and between 65 and 77 years to 22°. Therefore after age thirteen the range drops markedly and stabilises at about 30° from 35 to 64 and drops again to 20° after 65. About middle age the total range of lateral flexion is 60°, approximately equal to the total range of flexion and extension of the lumbar column. It is worthy of note that the segmental range of lateral flexion at L_5–S_1 is minimal as it rapidly drops from 7° in the child to 1° in the adult and to zero in the aged. The segmental range is maximal between L_3 and L_4, where it reaches 16° in the child, 8° in the adult and 6° in the aged.

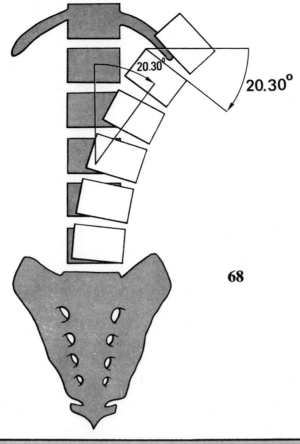

20.30°

20.30°

68

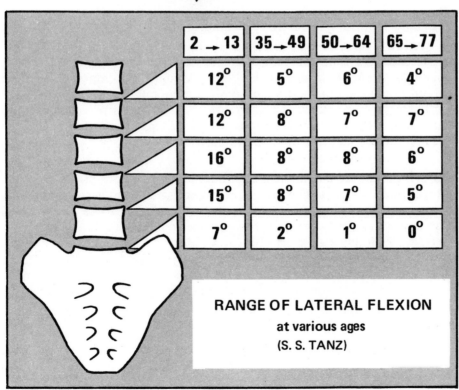

	2 → 13	35 → 49	50 → 64	65 → 77
	12°	5°	6°	4°
	12°	8°	7°	7°
	16°	8°	8°	6°
	15°	8°	7°	5°
	7°	2°	1°	0°

RANGE OF LATERAL FLEXION
at various ages
(S. S. TANZ)

69

RANGE OF ROTATION OF THE THORACOLUMBAR VERTEBRAL COLUMN

The range of rotation of the thoracolumbar column as a whole and at segmental level has been unknown for a long time. In fact, it is difficult to fix the pelvis and assess the rotation of the thoracic column because the free mobility of the shoulder girdle leaves a very wide margin for error. The recent work of Gregersen and Lucas has provided accurate measurements. Under general anaesthesia they implanted metal pins into the spinous processes of the thoracic and lumbar vertebrae and measured their displacements telemetrically. They were thus able to measure rotation of the thoracolumbar column during walking (fig. 70) and during standing and sitting (fig. 71).

During walking (fig. 70), it is clear (left part of graph) that the disc T_7–T_8 stays put while maximal rotation occurs at the discs immediately above and below (right part of graph). It is therefore next to this pivotal interspace that rotation has the greatest range, which then progressively decreases upwards and downwards to become minimal in the lumbar (0.3°) and upper thoracic (0.6°) regions.

In a study of the total range of rotation right and left (fig. 71), these authors show slight differences between the sitting and standing positions. In the sitting position the values are smaller as the pelvis is more easily fixed with the hips flexed. For the **lumbar column as a whole** the range of rotation is only 10°, i.e., an average of 1° per segment. For the thoracic column as a whole the range is appreciably greater, amounting to 75°, i.e., 37° on either side and about 3° for each segment. Therefore, despite the thoracic cage, rotation of the thoracic column is *four times greater* than that of the lumbar column. A comparison of the two curves reveals that both in the standing and sitting positions the total range of rotation to either side is the same. There are only qualitative differences between the two curves; for instance, the curve for standing has 4 points of inflexion, especially a point of inflexion in the lowest part of the lumbar region where rotation is more marked during standing, and a similar one at the zone of transition, i.e., the thoracolumbar joint.

In practice, it is impossible to implant electrodes into the spinous processes to study rotation and **clinical methods** are used. The subject is seated (fig. 72) and keeps the interscapular line fixed with respect to the thorax. He is then asked to rotate the trunk on either side and the range of rotation is measured as the angle between the interscapular line and the frontal plane. Here it is given as 15–20° but falls short of the maximum of 45° given by Gregersen and Lucas. A practical way of stabilising the interscapular line relative to the thorax is to rest the horizontally extended arms on to the handle of a broom placed across the back at scapular level. The interscapular line is then represented by the broom handle.

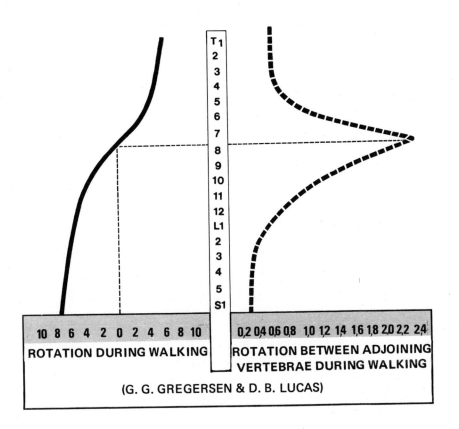

| ROTATION DURING WALKING | ROTATION BETWEEN ADJOINING VERTEBRAE DURING WALKING |

(G. G. GREGERSEN & D. B. LUCAS)

70

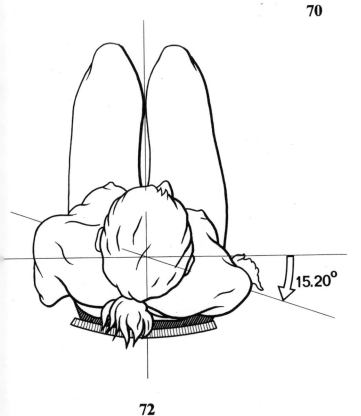

72

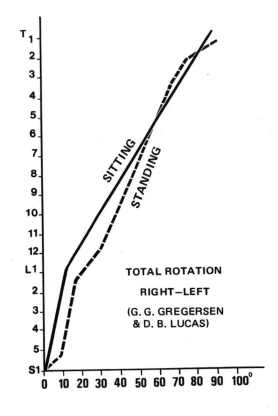

TOTAL ROTATION

RIGHT—LEFT

(G. G. GREGERSEN
& D. B. LUCAS)

71

119

THE INTERVERTEBRAL FORAMEN AND THE RADICULAR ORIFICE

It is impossible to complete this chapter on the functional anatomy of the lumbar vertebral column without a summary of the **physiopathology of nerve roots,** of particular importance in this region.

Some knowledge of anatomy is a prerequisite for the understanding of the diseases of nerve roots. Each nerve root (NR) leaves the vertebral canal through the **intervertebral foramen** (fig. 73). This foramen (2) is bounded by the posterior border of the *intervertebral disc* (I), the adjoining parts of the *vertebral bodies,* inferiorly and superiorly by the *pedicles* of the two adjoining vertebrae (10, 11) and posteriorly by the *articular processes and their joint* (9), which are linked by the capsular ligament (8) and the lateral edge of the *ligamentum flavum.* This ligament covers the joint capsule and encroaches upon the foramen.

Within the foramen the nerve root pierces the dura. Fig. 74 (seen in perspective) shows how the nerve root (NR), initially within the dura (3), approaches the internal aspect of the dura (4) and pierces it at a fixed point, i.e., **the radicular orifice** (5). The nerve must pass through this point where it is supported by the dura.

Fig. 75 (seen from above) shows again all these relations between the neuraxis and the vertebral canal. The spinal cord, surrounded by the dura (4), lies within the vertebral canal covered anteriorly by the posterior longitudinal ligament (12) and posteriorly by the ligamentum flavum (7). The anterior aspect of the joints between the articular processes (9) is lined by a capsule (8) reinforced by an extension of the ligamentum flavum (6). The nerve root, resting on the pedicle of the underlying vertebra (10), therefore passes through a narrow tunnel formed anteriorly by the disc and the posterior longitudinal ligament and posteriorly by the joint between the articular processes covered by an extension of the ligamentum flavum.

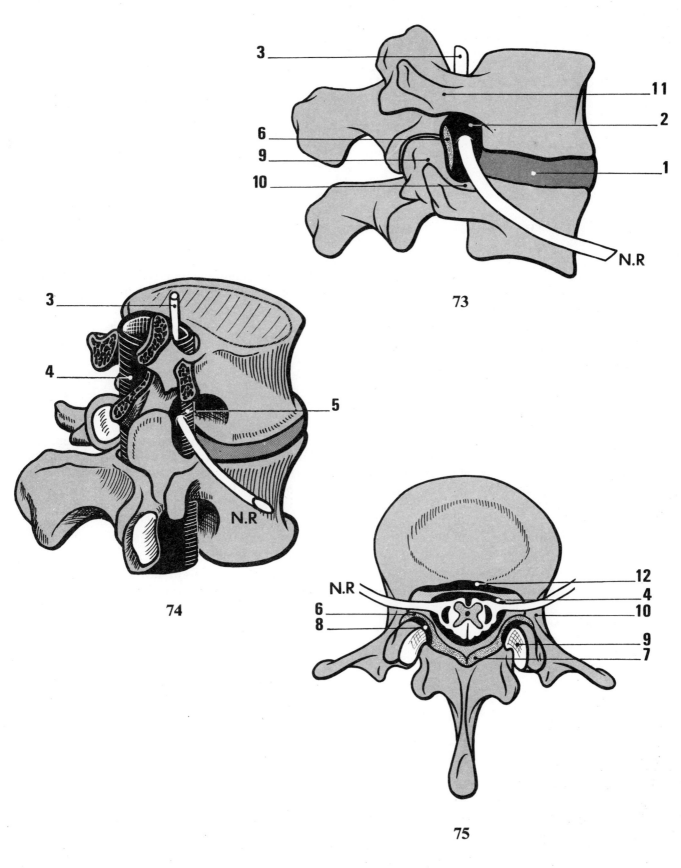

3

11

6
9
10

2

1

N.R

73

3

4

5

N.R

74

N.R

6
8

12
4
10

9
7

75

THE VARIOUS TYPES OF INTERVERTEBRAL DISC PROLAPSE

When compressed axially the substance of the nucleus pulposus can stream out in various directions. If the annulus is still strong the increase in pressure within the disc can cause the vertebral plateaus to give way. This corresponds to *intravertebral prolapse* (fig. 76).

Recent work has shown that the annulus fibres begin to degenerate after 25 years of age allowing tearing of fibres within each of its layers. Therefore under axial stress the nuclear material can stream out through the torn annulus (fig. 77). This streaming of nuclear material can be *concentric or more often radial*. Anterior prolapse is the rarest. Posterior prolapse is the most frequent, especially *posterolateral prolapse*. Thus, when the disc is crushed (fig. 78), part of the nuclear substance streams out anteriorly or more often posteriorly and can thus reach the posterior edge of the disc to touch the posterior longitudinal ligament (fig. 79). At first, the streamer, still *attached to the nucleus*, gets trapped under the posterior longitudinal ligament (A); in this case it is still possible to bring it back into its fibrous casing by vertebral traction. But very often it breaks through the posterior longitudinal ligament (B) and may lie within the vertebral canal—i.e., the so-called *free type of disc prolapse*. In other cases, the nuclear streamer is *trapped* under the posterior longitudinal ligament (C) and gets nipped off by the annulus fibres, which by snapping back into position preclude any restoration to normal. Finally, in some cases, the streamer, after reaching the deep aspect of the posterior longitudinal ligament, slides either superiorly or inferiorly (D). This is a case of *subligamentous prolapse*.

It is only when the herniating nucleus presses against the deep surface of the posterior longitudinal ligament that the nerve endings of the ligament are stretched causing *low back pain (lumbago)*. Finally compression of the nerve roots by the herniating disc causes *nerve root pain, i.e., sciatica*.

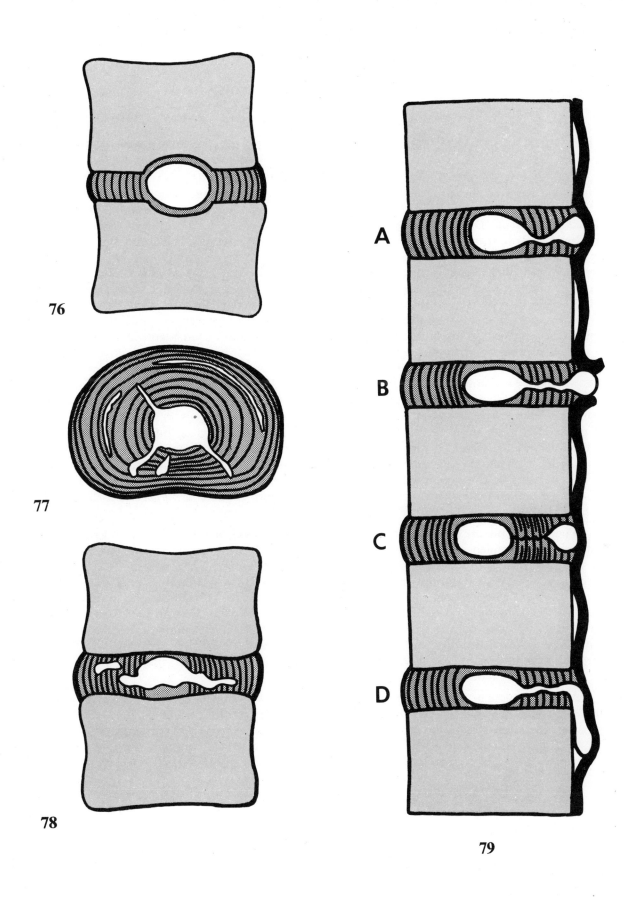

76

77

78

A

B

C

D

79

DISC PROLAPSE AND THE MECHANISM OF NERVE ROOT COMPRESSION

It is now generally believed that disc prolapse occurs in **three stages** (fig. 80). It only occurs if the disc has deteriorated as a result of *repeated microtraumas* and if the annulus fibres *have started to degenerate*. Disc prolapse usually follows *lifting of a weight with the trunk flexed forward*. **During the first stage** (A) trunk flexion flattens the discs anteriorly and opens out the inter-vertebral space posteriorly. **During the second stage** (B), *as soon as the weight is lifted*, the increased axial compression force crushes the whole disc and *violently drives the nuclear substance posteriorly* until it reaches the deep surface of the posterior longitudinal ligament. **During the third stage** (C) *with the trunk nearly straight*, the path taken by the herniating mass is closed by the pressure of the vertebral plateaus and the hernia remains trapped under the posterior longitudinal ligament. This causes the acute pain felt in the loin or lumbago which corresponds to the initial phase of the lumbago-sciatica complex. This initial acute lumbago can regress spontaneously or with treatment but, as a result of repeated trauma, the hernia grows in size and protrudes more and more into the vertebral canal. At this point it comes into contact with a nerve root, often *one of the nerve roots of the sciatic nerve* (fig. 81). In fact the hernia usually protrudes posterolaterally where the posterior longitudinal ligament is at its weakest and progressively pushes the nerve root away until the latter is jammed against the posterior wall of the intervertebral foramen formed by the joint between the articular processes, its anterior capsular ligament and the lateral border of the ligamentum flavum. From now on, the compressed nerve root will give rise to *pain* felt in the spinal segment corresponding to the root and finally to *impaired reflexes* (loss of the Achilles tendon reflex) and to *motor disturbances*, as in sciatica with paralysis.

The clinical picture (fig. 82) depends on the **spinal level** of disc prolapse and nerve root compression. If prolapse occurs at L_4–L_5 (1) the root of L_5 is compressed and pain is felt in the posterolateral aspect of the thigh, the knee, the lateral border of the calf, the lateral border of the instep of the foot and the dorsal surface of the foot down to the big toe. If the prolapse lies at L_5–S_1 (2), S_1 is compressed and pain is referred to the posterior aspect of the thigh, knee and calf, the heel and the lateral border of the foot down to the fifth toe. However, this correlation of clinical picture and lesion level is not absolute. For example, a hernia at L_4–L_5 may lie closer to the midline and compress at once L_5 and S_1 or even occasionally S_1 alone. Surgical exploration at L_5–S_1, done on the strength of the S_1 root pain, may fail to recognise the lesion that lies at one level above.

A sagittal section (fig. 82) slightly modifies the view obtained on the transverse section (fig. 81), which shows the presence of the spinal cord. In fact the cord stops at L_2 to become the conus medullaris. Below the conus the dura contains only the nerve roots arranged in horse tail fashion (cauda equina) and they emerge two by two at each level through the intervertebral foramen. At L_4–L_5 level there are still four root pairs in the dura; at L_5–S_1 level the L_5 roots have already left and there are only three remaining nerve root pairs. The dura ends as a cul-de-sac at S_3 (D).

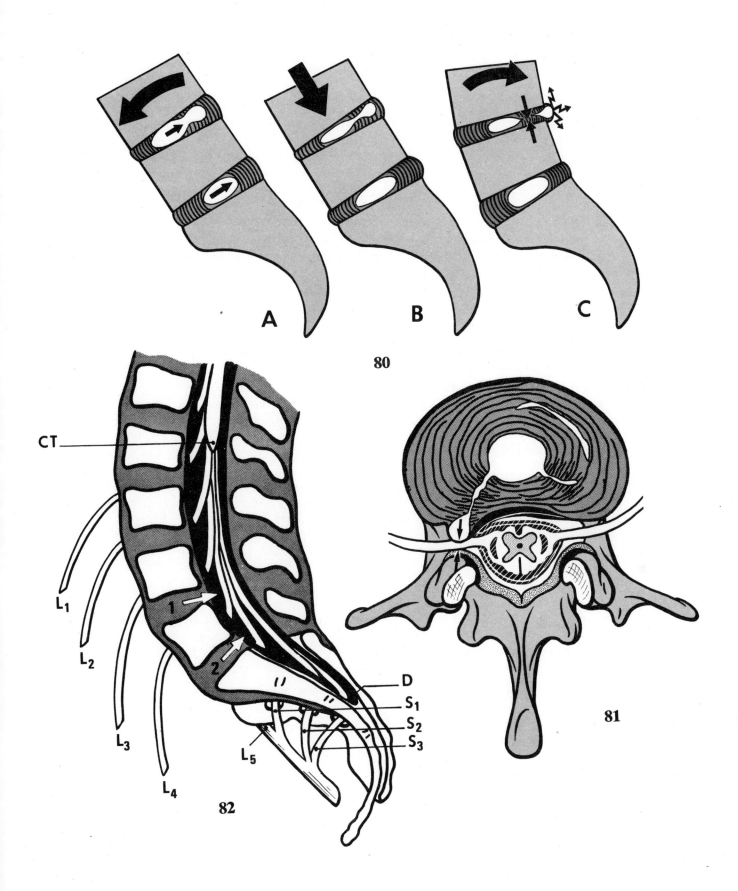

A

B

C

80

CT

L₁

L₂

L₃

L₄

1

2

L₅

D

S₁

S₂

S₃

82

81

125

LASÈGUE'S SIGN

Lasègue's sign is the pain induced by *stretching the sciatic nerve* or one of its roots. It is elicited by gradual and slow elevation of the extended lower limb with the subject supine. The pain induced is similar to that felt spontaneously by the subject, i.e., in the same area of distribution.

Charnley has shown that the *nerve roots glide freely through the intervertebral foramina* and that, during elevation of the extended lower limb, the nerve roots are pulled out of the foramina for a distance of up to 12 mm at L_5 level (fig. 87).

Lasègue's sign can therefore be interpreted as follows:

when the subject is supine, with the lower limbs resting on the supporting surface (fig. 83), the sciatic nerve and its roots are under no tension;

when the lower limb is raised *with the knees flexed* (fig. 84) the sciatic nerve and its roots are still under no tension;

but if the lower limb is elevated *with the knee extended* (fig. 85) the sciatic nerve, which must cover a longer distance, is subjected to increasing tension. In the normal person the nerve roots slide freely through the intervertebral foramina and no pain results, but, when the lower limb is nearly vertical, pain is felt on the posterior aspect of the thigh as a result of stretching the hamstrings in people with diminished flexibility. This ia a *false positive Lasègue sign*;

on the other hand, when one nerve root is trapped in the foramen or when it must cover a longer distance because of a prolapsed disc, any stretching of the nerve will become painful with moderate elevation of the lower limb. This is a *positive Lasègue sign*, which generally is evident before 60° flexion is attained. In fact, after 60° flexion, the Lasègue sign is not applicable since the sciatic nerve achieves maximal tension at 60° flexion. Thus pain may be elicited at 10°, 15° or 20° flexion and this allows a rough quantitation of the severity of the lesion.

One point deserves emphasis. During forced elevation of the limb with extended knee the force of traction on the nerve roots can reach 3 kg. Now the resistance to traction of these nerve roots is 3.2 kg. Therefore if a root is trapped or relatively shortened by a prolapsed disc, any rough manipulation of the leg can cause *rupture of some axons* which may result in *paralysis*. This is usually shortlived but occasionally may take a long time to disappear. Therefore two precautions must be observed:

on the one hand, *one must always elicit the Lasègue sign gently and cautiously* and stop when pain is felt;

on the other hand, *one must never elicit the sign under general anaesthesia* since the protective pain reflex is absent. This can occur when the patient is being placed prone on the operating table and the hips are allowed to flex with the knees extended. The surgeon must always *personally* place the patient on the table and make sure that hip flexion *is always associated with knee flexion*, which relaxes the sciatic nerve and the trapped root.

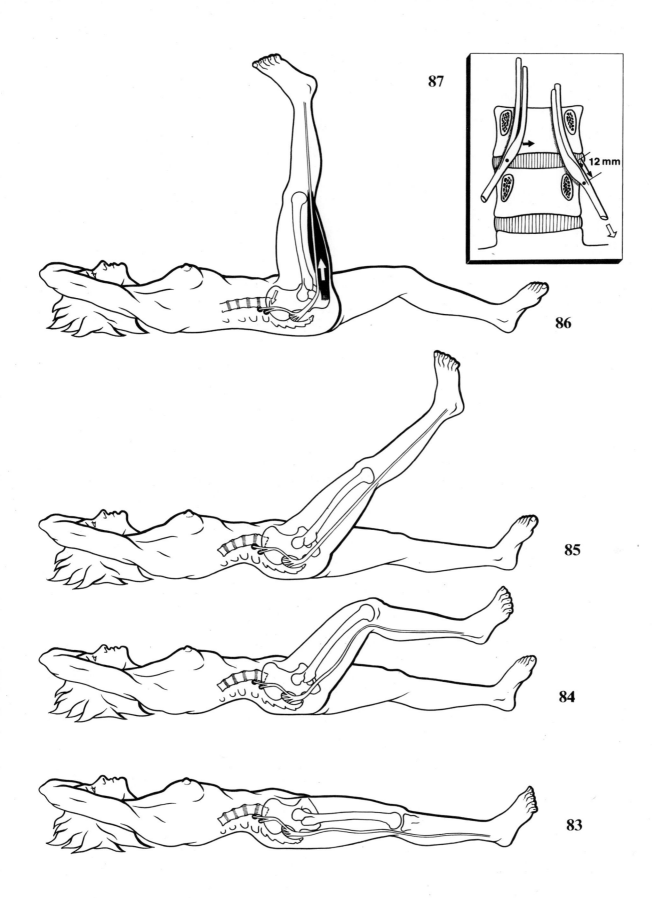

87

12 mm

86

85

84

83

THE THORACIC VERTEBRAL COLUMN

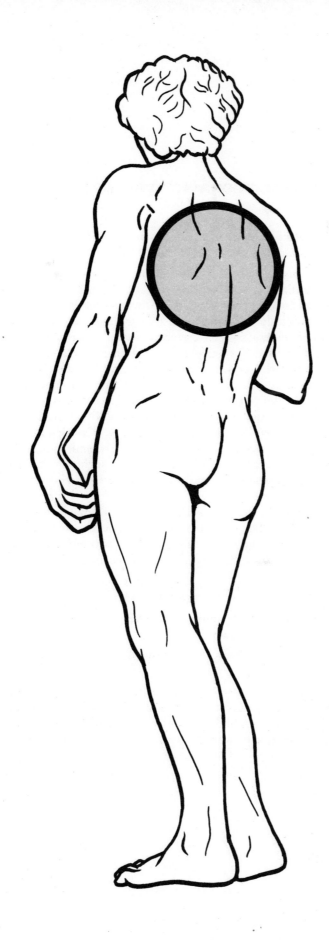

THE TYPICAL THORACIC VERTEBRA AND T_{12}

The **typical thoracic vertebra** (fig. 2) is made up of the same parts as a lumbar vertebra but with important structural and functional differences.

Fig. 1 (the vertebra has been 'exploded') shows the *vertebral body* (1) with roughly equal transverse and anteroposterior diameters. It is proportionately higher than the lumbar vertebra and its anterior and lateral surfaces are quite hollow. The posterolateral corner of the vertebral plateau bears an oval articular facet, obliquely set and lined by cartilage; this is the *costal articular facet* which will be discussed later in relation to costovertebral joints. Posterolaterally the vertebral body bears the *two pedicles* (2 and 3) and the superior costal facet often extends into the root of the pedicle. Posterior to the pedicles arise *the laminae* (4 and 5), which form the greater part of the vertebral arch. These laminae are higher than they are wide and are set obliquely like tiles on a roof; near the pedicle their superior border gives attachment to the *superior articular processes* (6 and 7), which bear an articular facet. This cartilage-lined facet is oval, flat or slightly convex transversely and *faces posteriorly, slightly superiorly and slightly laterally*. On the inferior border of the lamina, still near the pedicle, lies the *inferior articular process* (only the right one is seen here, 8), which has an articular facet on its anterior surface. This cartilage-lined facet is oval, plane or slightly concave transversely and *faces anteriorly, slightly inferiorly and medially*; it is connected to the superior articular process of the overlying vertebra. To the junction of lamina and pedicle near the articular process is attached the *transverse process* (9 and 11), facing laterally and slightly posteriorly. It has a bulbous tip which bears on its anterior aspect a *small articular facet* (10) corresponding to the costal tubercle. The two laminae meet in the midline to form the long and bulky *spinous process* (12), which is sharply inclined inferiorly and posteriorly and has a single tubercle on its tip.

When these elements are put together the typical thoracic vertebra is formed (fig. 2).

The last thoracic vertebra (T_{12}), acting as a *bridge* between the thoracic and lumbar regions, has certain characteristics of its own:

first, its body has only two costal facets for the twelfth ribs, located at the posterolateral angle of the *vertebral plateau*;

next, while its superior articular processes resemble those of the other thoracic vertebrae in facing posteriorly and slightly superiorly and laterally, the inferior articular processes must correspond to those of L_1. Therefore, like those of the lumbar vertebrae, they *face laterally and anteriorly* and are slightly convex transversely with their centres of curvature lying roughly at the origin of the spinous process.

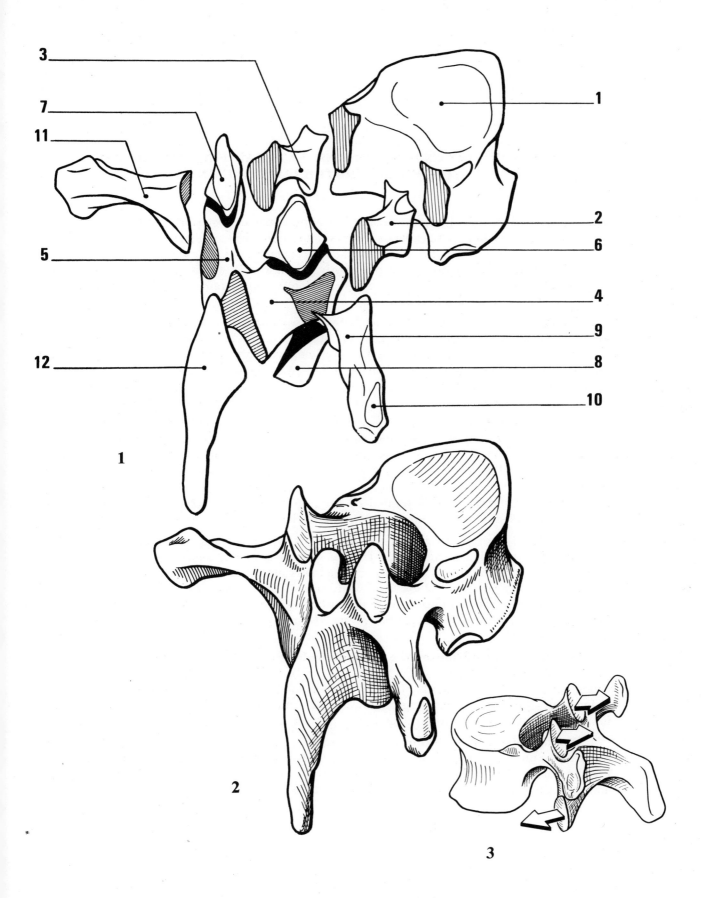

3

7

11

5

12

1

1

2

6

4

9

8

10

2

3

FLEXION AND EXTENSION AND LATERAL FLEXION OF THE THORACIC VERTEBRAL COLUMN

During extension (fig. 4) the vertebrae are approximated posteriorly and crush the disc posteriorly. As a result the disc expands anteriorly and the nucleus pulposus is driven anteriorly. Extension is limited by the *impact of the articular processes* (1) and *the spinous processes* (2) which, being sharply inclined inferiorly and posteriorly, are normally almost touching. The *anterior longitudinal ligament* is stretched while the posterior longitudinal ligament, the ligamenta flava and the interspinous ligaments are relaxed.

Duing flexion (fig. 5) the interspace between two vertebrae opens out posteriorly and the nucleus is displaced posteriorly. The articular surfaces of the articular processes slide upward and the inferior articular processes of the overlying vertebra tend to overhang the superior processes of the underlying vertebra. Flexion is limited by *the tension developed in the interspinous ligament* (4), *the ligamenta flava, the capsular ligaments of the joints between the articular processes* (5) *and the posterior longitudinal ligament*; conversely, the anterior longitudinal ligament is relaxed.

During lateral flexion (fig. 6, seen from the back) the articular facets of the articular processes of any two adjacent vertebrae slide relative to each other. On the contralateral side the facets slide as in flexion, i.e., upwards; on the ipsilateral side they slide as in extension, i.e., downwards. The line joining the two transverse processes of the upper vertebra mm′ and the corresponding line in the lower vertebra nn′ form an angle equivalent to the angle of lateral flexion. Lateral flexion is limited by the impact of the articular processes on the side of movement and also by the contralateral ligamenta flava and intertransverse ligaments.

It would be incorrect to discuss the movements of the thoracic vertebral column only in relation to the individual vertebrae. In fact *the thoracic column is connected to the thoracic cage by multiple joints* (fig. 7) and all the·bony, cartilaginous and articular components of the cage play a role in *orienting and limiting the basic movement of the column*. Thus, in the skeleton, the thoracic column by itself is more mobile than when it is still connected with the thoracic cage. Therefore one must study the *changes in the thoracic cage associated with movements of the thoracic column*.

During lateral flexion of the thoracic column (fig. 8), on the contralateral side the thorax is elevated (1), the intercostal spaces widen (3), the thoracic cage is enlarged (5) and the chondrocostal angle of the tenth rib tends to open out (7). On the ipsilateral side the opposite changes are seen: the thoracic cage is lowered (2) and shrinks (6), the intercostal spaces are narrowed (4) and the chondrocostal angle becomes smaller (8).

During flexion of the thoracic column (fig. 9), all the angles between the various segments of the thorax and between the thorax and vertebral column open out, i.e., the costo-vertebral angle (1), the superior (2) and inferior (3) sternocostal angles and the chondrocostal angle (4). Conversely during extension all these angles become smaller.

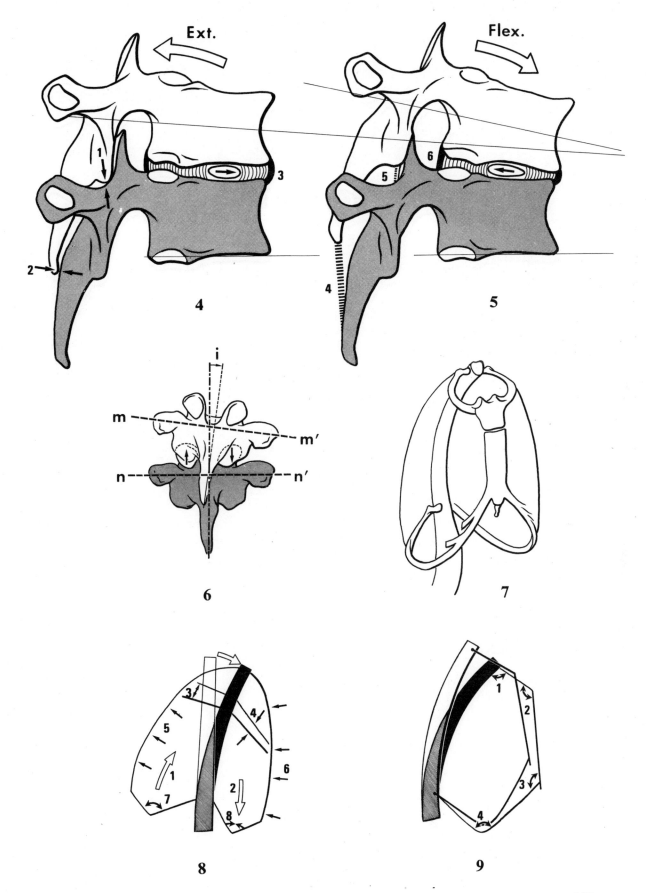

Ext.

Flex.

4

5

6

7

8

9

AXIAL ROTATION OF THE THORACIC VERTEBRAL COLUMN

The mechanism of axial rotation at thoracic level differs from that seen at lumbar level. In fact (fig. 10), the joints between the articular processes have a completely different orientation. The profile of the interspace also corresponds to *the surface of a cylinder but the centre of this cylinder lies more or less at the centre of each vertebral body*. When one vertebra rotates on another, the articular facets of the articular processes slide relative to each other and this leads to rotation of a vertebral body relative to another about this common axis. This is followed by rotation and twisting of the intervertebral disc and not by shearing movements of the disc as in the lumbar region. This rotation and twisting of the disc has a greater range of movement, especially as the elementary rotation of a thoracic vertebra is at least three times that of a lumbar vertebra.

However, this rotation would be greater if the thoracic column was not intimately connected with the bony thorax. In fact, *any movement at each level of the column induces a similar movement in the corresponding ribs* (fig. 11) but the sliding of a rib pair on the underlying pair is limited by *the presence of the sternum* to which each rib is attached by a costal cartilage. Therefore rotation of a vertebra will lead to distortion of the corresponding rib pair owing to the elasticity of the rib, especially of its cartilage. These distortions are as follows:

accentuation of the concavity of the rib on the side of vertebral rotation (1);

flattening of the concavity of the rib on the opposite side (2);

accentuation of the chondrocostal concavity on the side opposite to vertebral rotation (3);

flattening of the concavity of the chondrocostal angle on the side of rotation.

During this movement the sternum is subject to shearing forces and it comes to lie obliquely superoinferiorly so as to follow the rotation of the vertebral bodies. This induced obliquity of the sternum is very small and cannot be shown clinically; radiologically it is difficult to demonstrate because of superimposition of multiple planes.

The mechanical resistance of the thorax therefore plays a role in limiting appreciably the range of movement of the thoracic column. When the thorax is still flexible, as in the young, the movements of the thoracic column have a considerable range but with age the costal cartilages ossify and this reduces the chondrocostal elasticity. As a result, in the aged the thorax is almost rigid and movement is correspondingly reduced.

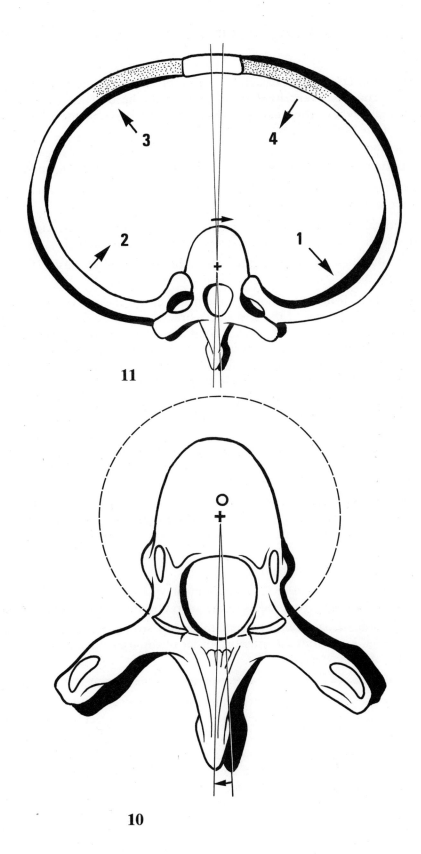

11

10

135

THE COSTOVERTEBRAL JOINTS

At each level of the thoracic vertebral column a pair of ribs is connected with a vertebra by means of two joints: **the costovertebral joint** between the head of the rib, the intervertebral disc and the vertebral bodies; **the costo-transverse joint** between the rib tubercle and the transverse process of the underlying vertebra.

Fig. 12 (taken obliquely) shows one rib removed and some ligaments resected so as to reveal the vertebral articular surfaces; the underlying rib is left in place with its ligaments.

Fig. 13 (seen from above) shows the right rib in position but the joints have been opened; the left rib has been removed after section of its ligaments.

Fig. 14 (a vertical section in the frontal plane) passes through the right costovertebral joint; on the left side the rib has been removed after section of its ligaments.

We shall describe these joints using the three figures simultaneously (the numbers are common to all the figures).

The **costovertebral joint** is a synovial joint made up on the vertebral side by two costal facets, one on the superior border of the lower vertebra (5) and the other on the inferior border of the upper vertebra (6). These facets form a solid angle (easily seen in fig. 14), whose base consists of the annulus fibrosus of the intervertebral disc. The corresponding facets of the head of the rib (12) are slightly convex and also form between each other a solid angle which fits exactly into the angle formed by the costal facets of the vertebrae.

An interosseous ligament (8), attached to the head of the rib between the two articular facets and to the intervertebral disc, divides this joint, surrounded by a *single capsule*, into two distinct cavities, superior and inferior (13). The costovertebral joint is reinforced by a *radiate ligament* consisting of three bands: *a superior band* (14), and *an inferior band* (15) attached to the adjacent vertebral bodies and *an intermediate band* (16) inserted into the annulus fibrosus of the intervertebral disc.

The costotransverse joint is also a *synovial joint* consisting of two oval articular facets, the one *on the tip of the transverse process* (18) and the *other on the costal tubercle* (19). It is surrounded by a *capsule* (20) but above all it is strengthened by three costotransverse ligaments:

the interosseous costotransverse ligament (23), very short and strong, runs from the transverse process to the posterior surface of the neck of the rib;

the posterior costotransverse ligament (21), rectangular in shape, 1.5 cm long and 1 cm wide, runs from the tip of the transverse process to the lateral border of the costal tubercle;

the superior costotransverse ligament (24), very thick and strong, flat and quadrilateral, 8 mm wide and 10 mm long, runs from the inferior border of the transverse process to the superior border of the neck of the underlying rib.

Some authors also describe *an inferior costotransverse ligament* underlying the joint.

In these figures one can see again the details of the intervertebral disc with the nucleus pulposus (1), the annulus fibrosus (2), the joints between the articular processes with their articular facets (3) and their capsules (4).

On the whole, the rib is connected to the vertebral column by **two synovial joints**: a simple joint, the costotransverse; a double joint, more solidly interlocked, the costovertebral. These joints are reinforced by strong ligaments.

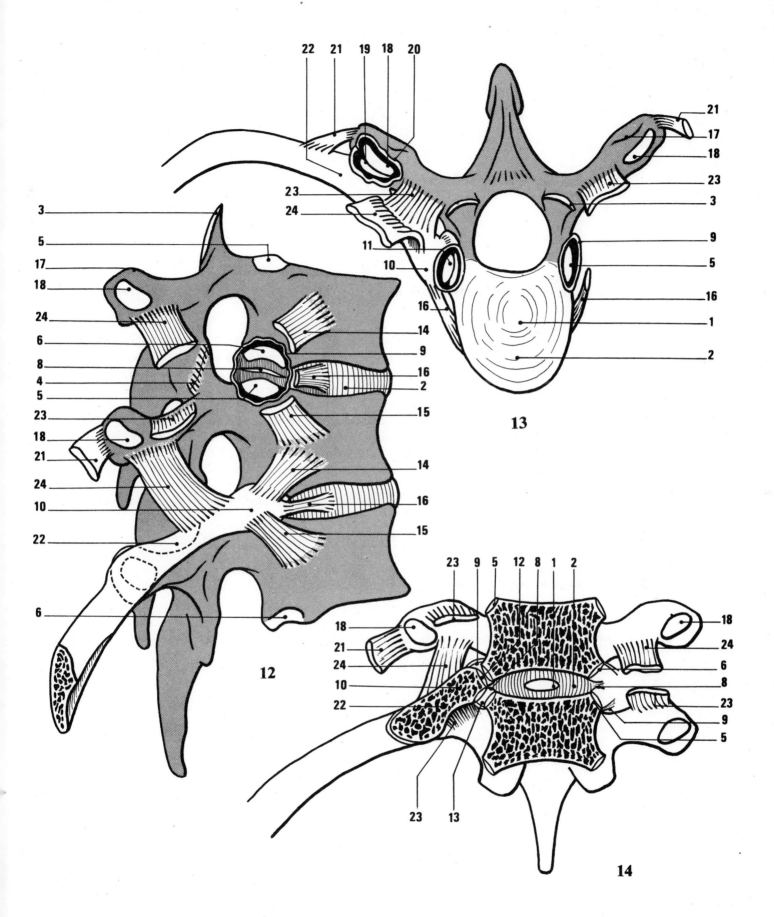

MOVEMENTS OF THE RIBS AT THE COSTOVERTEBRAL JOINTS

The costovertebral joint, on the one hand, and the costotransverse, on the other, form a *joint couple mechanically linked* (fig. 15), whose common movement can only be *rotation about an axis passing through the centre of each joint*. This axis XX′, running through the centre O of the costotransverse joint and the centre O′ of the costovertebral joint, acts as a swivel for the rib, which is thus 'suspended' from the vertebral column at two points O and O′. The direction of this axis with respect to the sagittal plane determines the direction of movement of the rib. For the **lower ribs** (left side of the figure) the axis xx′ lies nearly parallel to the sagittal plane and so elevation of the rib increases the transverse diameter of the thorax by a distance l. In fact (fig. 17), when the rib rotates about this axis, it describes an arc of a circle with centre O: it becomes less oblique and more transverse and as a result its most lateral border moves laterally over a distance l, which represents the increase in the transverse diameter of the thoracic outlet.

On the other hand, the axis yy′ for the **upper ribs** (fig. 15: right side) lies closer to the frontal plane. Therefore elevation of these ribs increases the anteroposterior diameter of the thorax by a distance a. In effect (fig. 16), when the anterior end of the rib is raised by a distance h, it describes an arc of a circle and is displaced anteriorly by a distance a.

It follows, therefore, that elevation of the ribs *increases the transverse diameter of the lower thorax and the anteroposterior diameter of the upper thorax*. In the midzone, the costovertebral joints have an axis lying obliquely at an angle of 45° to the sagittal plane so that both diameters are increased.

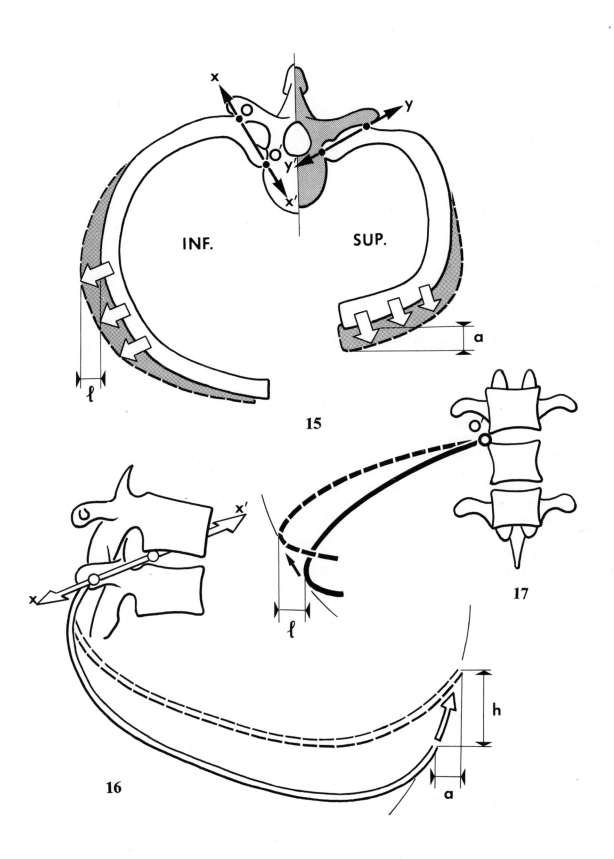

INF.

SUP.

a

ℓ

15

16

17

h

a

ℓ

MOVEMENTS OF THE COSTAL CARTILAGES AND OF THE STERNUM

So far only the movements of the ribs at the costovertebral and costotransverse joints have been considered but rib movements relative to the sternum and costal cartilages must also be taken into account. If these movements are viewed from above (fig. 18) and from the front (fig. 19) it is clear that, whereas the *most lateral part of the rib is raised* by a distance h′ and is pushed laterally by a distance l, the anterior end of the rib is raised by a distance h and is pushed anteriorly by a distance l′ (h = h′ and l′ = l). At the same time, the *sternum is raised* and the costal cartilage becomes more horizontal forming an angle a with its initial position. *This angular movement of the costal cartilage* relative to the sternum occurs at the *sternocostal joint.* Simultaneously another movement occurs at the costochondral junction, which will be discussed later.

When the rib is raised (fig. 18: right side), the point of maximum increase in thoracic diameter is the point most distant from the axis xx′. This geometrical fact explains how this point varies from rib to rib with changes in the obliquity of their axes.

140

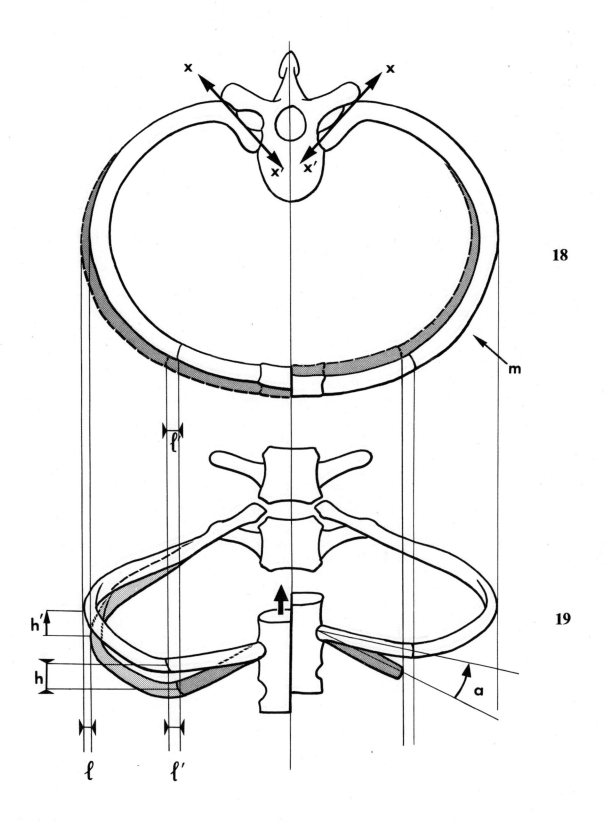

18

19

141

THE SHAPE CHANGES OF THE THORAX IN THE SAGITTAL PLANE DURING INSPIRATION

Supposing that the vertebral column is fixed during inspiration (fig. 20), one need only consider the changes in shape of the flexible pentagon formed, on the one hand, by the vertebral column and, on the other, by the first rib, the sternum, the tenth rib and its costal cartilage. These changes are as follows:

the first rib, being freely mobile about its costovertebral joint (O), is elevated so that its anterior end describes an *arc of a circle* AA′;

as the first rib is elevated *so is the sternum* which moves from AB to A′B′;

during this movement the *sternum does not stay parallel to its initial position* as the antero-posterior diameter of the upper thorax is increased more than that of the lower thorax. It follows that the angle between the sternum and the vertical (a) becomes slightly more acute and the angle OA′B′ is smaller than the initial angle OAB. The sternocostal angle is reduced as a result of axial rotation of the costal cartilage (see page 162);

the tenth rib is also raised, with Q as its centre of rotation, and its anterior end describes an arc of a circle CC′;

as both the tenth rib and the sternum are raised the tenth costal cartilage moves from CB to a roughly parallel position C′B′. It follows that the angle C′ is greater than the angle C by a value c which is equal to the angle C′QC—the angle of elevation of the tenth rib. The chondrocostal angle C′B′A′ is also greater than the original angle CBA. Once more, this widening of the angle is achieved by axial rotation of the cartilage. A similar axial rotation takes place in all the costal cartilages. We shall see later the role this has to play in maintaining the elasticity of the thorax.

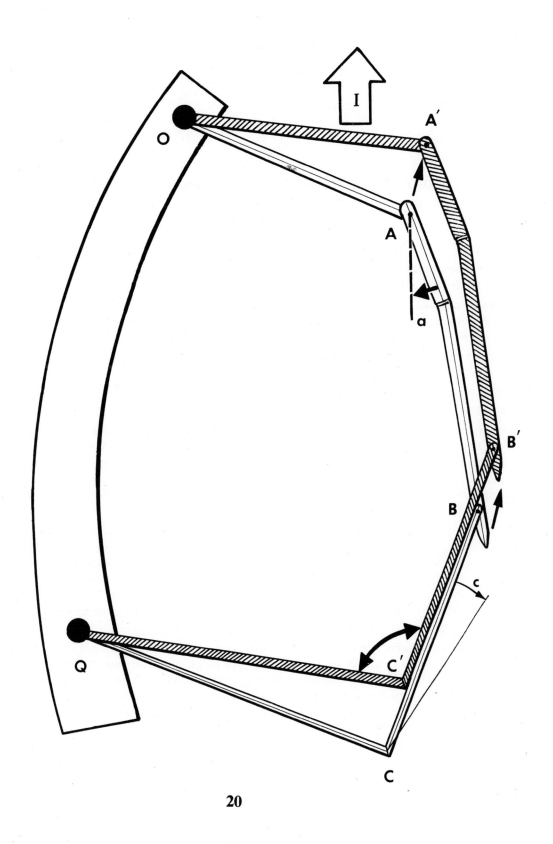

20

MODE OF ACTION OF THE INTERCOSTAL MUSCLES
AND THE STERNOCOSTALIS

A posterior view of the thorax and the vertebral column (fig. 21) shows three sets of muscles:

the **levator costae** (L), attached to the tip of the transverse process and the superior border of the rib below, acts by *elevating the rib*;

the **external intercostal muscle** (E), with its fibres running parallel to the levator costae as they course obliquely superiorly and medially. Therefore this muscle and the levator *elevate* ribs and act as *inspiratory* muscles;

the **internal intercostal muscle** (I), with its oblique fibres running superiorly and laterally, *depresses the ribs* and so is an *expiratory* muscle.

The mode of action of these muscles is well explained by these diagrams (according to Hamberger):

the action of the *external intercostal* (fig. 22) is easily grasped if one realises that the direction of its fibres is parallel to the long diagonal of the parallelogram OO'BA formed by the ribs connected to the vertebral column and the sternum. When the muscle contracts (E) the diagonal is shortened by a distance r and this distorts the parallelogram. Assuming that OO' is fixed, this causes rotation of A_1 to A_2 and B_1 to B_2. Therefore contraction of the external intercostal *elevates the ribs* and the muscle is a *muscle of inspiration*;

the action of the *internal intercostal* (fig. 23) can be understood in a similar way except that the direction of the muscle fibres is parallel to the short diagonal of the parallelogram. When the muscle (I) contracts, the diagonal OA' is shortened by a distance r' which displaces A_1 to A_2 and B_1 to B_2, assuming that OO' is fixed. The internal intercostal therefore *depresses the ribs* and *is active in expiration*. This demonstration of Hamberger was at one time contradicted by Duchenne de Boulogne's electrical stimulation experiments but more recent electromyographic studies have supported it.

The **sternocostalis** is a small muscle which is usually ignored because of its retro-sternal location (fig. 24). It lies entirely on the deep surface of the sternum and its fibres, inserted into the second to sixth ribs, run obliquely inferiorly and medially. Contraction of its five muscle bands *depresses the corresponding costal cartilages relative to the sternum*. We have seen (fig. 19) that the costal cartilage is raised during inspiration and depressed during expiration; the sternocostalis, therefore, is a *muscle of expiration*.

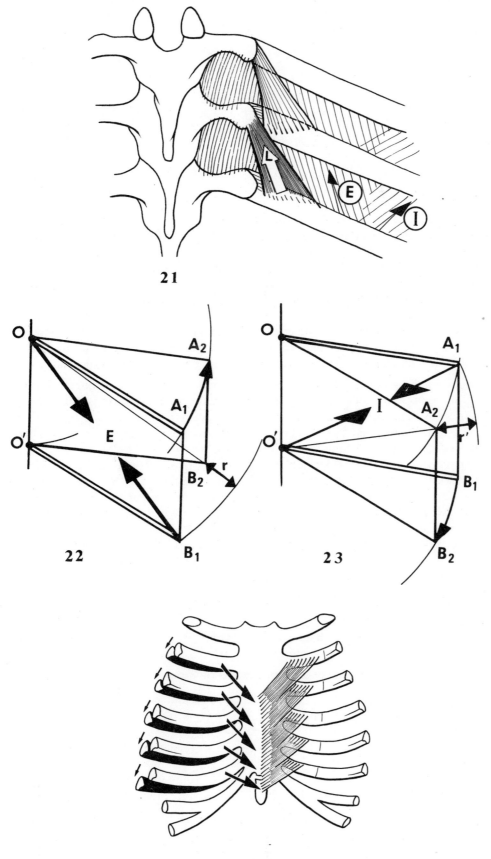

21

22

23

24

THE DIAPHRAGM AND ITS MODE OF ACTION

The diaphragm is a *musculo-tendinous dome forming the floor of the thorax and separating the thorax and abdomen*. Seen from the side (fig. 25) this dome reaches farther down posteriorly than anteriorly and its apex is the central tendon (1). From this centre, bands of muscle fibres (2) radiate out to the periphery of the floor of the thorax and gain attachment to the deep surfaces of the costal cartilages, the tips of the eleventh and twelfth ribs, the costal arch, the vertebral bodies by means of crura (left crus 3 and right crus 4), the medial surfaces of the psoas (7) and the quadratus lumborum (8). This is more obvious when seen from in front (fig. 26), where it is easy to distinguish at the same time the apex of the diaphragm and its inner surface at the level of the crura. The openings in the diaphragm can also be seen as they allow the passage of the oesophagus (6) and the aorta (5). In this figure the opening for the inferior vena cava is not shown.

When the diaphragm contracts the *central tendon is pulled down* thus increasing the vertical diameter of the thorax. One can therefore compare the diaphragm to a piston sliding inside a pump. This depression of the central tendon is rapidly checked by the mediastinal constituents as they are stretched, and by the resistance offered by the abdominal organs. From this moment on (fig. 27) the central tendon becomes fixed (large white arrow) and the muscle fibres, now acting from the periphery of this central tendon (small white arrow), elevate the lower ribs. In effect, if one considers P as fixed and the rib as rotating about an axis O, the rib extremity describes an arc of a circle AB while the corresponding muscle fibres shorten by a distance of A'B. Therefore by elevating the lower ribs the *diaphragm increases the transverse diameter of the lower thorax* and simultaneously, with the help of the sternum, it also elevates the upper ribs, *thus increasing also the anteroposterior diameter of the thorax*. Therefore the diaphragm can be considered as the basic muscle of respiration as **it increases by itself all three diameters of the thoracic cavity**:

it increases the vertical diameter by pulling down the central tendon;

it increases the transverse diameter by elevating the lower ribs;

it increases the anteroposterior diameter by elevating the upper ribs with the help of the sternum;

Its significance in the physiology of respiration is obvious.

146

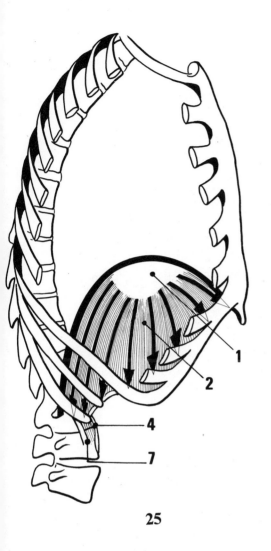

25

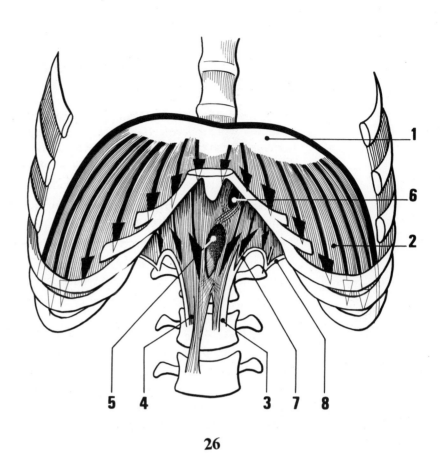

26

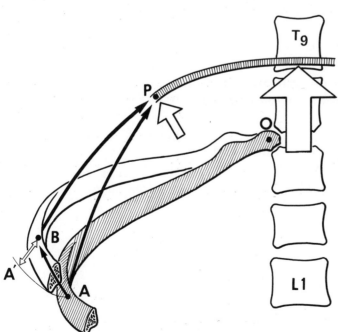

27

147

THE RESPIRATORY MUSCLES

From the foregoing, one can divide respiratory muscles into two groups: the **inspiratory muscles** which *elevate the ribs* and the **expiratory muscles** which *depress the ribs and the sternum*. These groups can be subdivided into two groups—the *primary* and the *accessory muscles*, the latter being recruited only when respiratory movements are unusually deep or strong.

These muscles can therefore be divided into four groups:

Group I: the **primary inspiratory** muscles—the external intercostals, the sternocostalis and above all the **diaphragm**.

Group II: the **accessory muscles of inspiration** (fig. 28, 29, 30):

the sternomastoid (1), the scalenus anterior (2), medius (3) and posterior (4) only help in inspiration when they can act on a cervical vertebral column fixed by other muscles (fig. 28);

the pectoralis major (4) and minor (5) when they act on the scapula and upper limb already in abduction;

the inferior fibres of the serratus anterior (5) and the latissimus dorsi (10), when the latter acts on the upper limb already in abduction;

the serratus posterior superior (11);

the superior fibres of the iliocostalis (12) which are attached superiorly to the last five cervical transverse processes and inferiorly to the first six costal arches. It resembles the levator costae in the direction of its fibres.

Group III: the primary expiratory muscles—the internal intercostals. In fact *normal expiration is a purely passive process due* to recoil of the thorax as a result of the *elasticity* of its osteochondral components and of the pulmonary parenchyma. The energy necessary for expiration derives from the energy developed by the inspiratory muscles and stored by the elastic components of the thorax and lungs. We shall see later the essential role played by the costal cartilages. Let us note also that during standing the ribs are pulled by their own weights and thus the *contribution of gravity* is not negligible.

Group IV: the **accessory expiratory muscles**. Though accessory, they are no less important and they are extremely powerful. They allow **forced expiration** and the **performance of the Valsalva manoeuvre**.

The abdominal muscles (fig. 30), the rectus abdominis (7), the external oblique (8), the internal oblique (9) strongly depress the thoracic floor.

In the thoracolumbar region (fig. 29) other accessory muscles are present: the lowest fibres of the iliocostalis (13), the longissimus (14), the serratus posterior inferior (15) and the quadratus lumborum (not shown here).

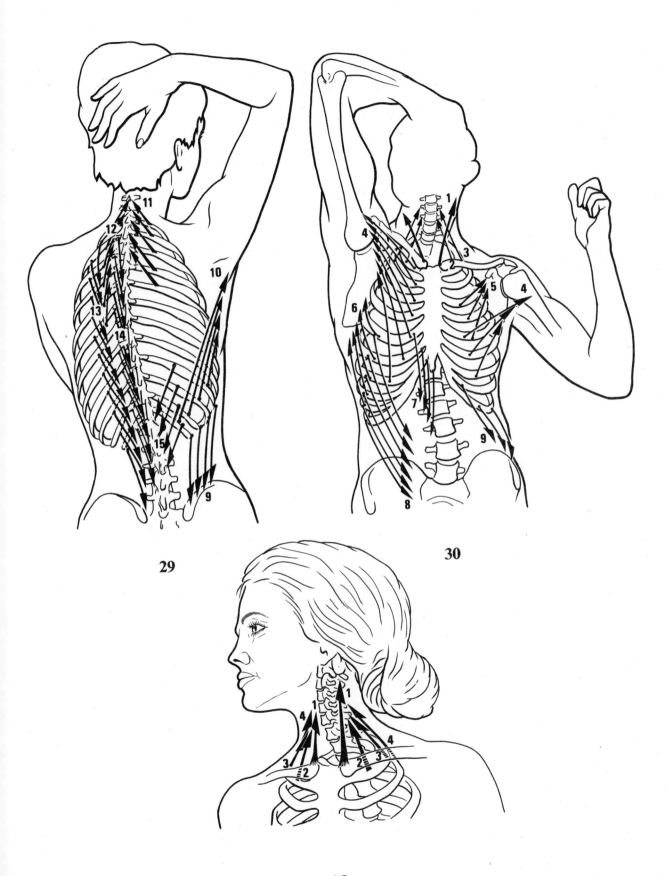

29

30

28

ANTAGONISM AND SYNERGISM OF THE DIAPHRAGM AND THE ABDOMINAL MUSCLES

As already shown, the diaphragm is the main inspiratory muscle and the abdominal muscles are accessory expiratory muscles of great strength, which can produce forced expiration. *Though apparently antagonistic these muscles are also synergistic.* In fact the diaphragm would be less effective in the absence of the abdominal muscles.

During inspiration (fig. 31: seen from the side; fig. 32: seen from the front) the contraction of the diaphragm brings down the central tendon increasing the vertical diameter of the thorax; but this is soon opposed by the elongation of the vertical mediastinal elements (M) and especially the *resistance of the abdominal viscera* (D). These are contained within the 'abdominal girdle' formed by the powerful abdominal muscles: the rectus muscles (R), the transversus muscles (T), the internal (IO) and external obliquus (EO). Without these muscles, the abdominal contents would be displaced inferiorly and anteriorly and the central tendon would not be stabilised to allow the diaphragm to elevate the lower ribs. *This antagonistic–synergistic action of the abdominal muscles therefore is essential for the efficiency of the diaphragm.* This is borne out in disease, e.g., in poliomyelitis, where the paralysis of the abdominal muscles reduces the ventilatory efficiency of the diaphragm. In fig. 31 (seen from the side) the directions of the fibres of the abdominal muscles represent a six-sided star.

During expiration (fig. 33: seen from the side; fig. 34: seen from in front) the diaphragm relaxes and contraction of the abdominal muscles lowers the thoracic floor thereby decreasing simultaneously the transverse and anteroposterior diameters of the thorax. Also by increasing the intra-abdominal pressure they push the viscera upwards and raise the central tendon. This decreases the vertical diameter of the thorax and 'closes' the costodiaphragmatic recesses. Therefore the abdominal muscles are the *perfect antagonists of the diaphragm* as they reduce simultaneously the three diameters of the thorax.

The respective roles of the diaphragm and abdominal muscles can be visualised as follows (fig. 35). Both sets of muscles are always in active contraction but their activity varies reciprocally. Thus, during inspiration the tonus of the diaphragm increases while that of the abdominal muscles decreases, and vice versa during expiration. Hence there exists between these two muscle groups a *floating equilibrium* constantly shifting in both directions; this is the basis of the antagonism–synergism of these muscles.

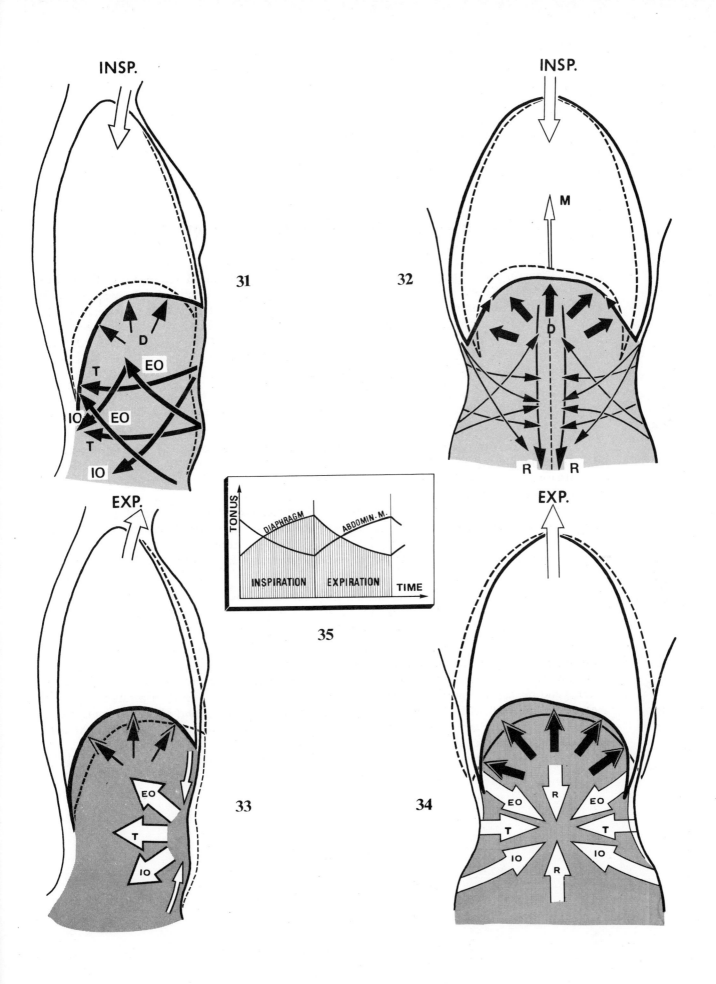

AIR MOVEMENT IN THE RESPIRATORY AIRWAYS

Air movement in the bronchial tree is demonstrated by the **classical experiment of Funck** (figs. 36 and 37). Replace the bottom of a flask by a watertight elastic membrane and insert inside the flask a balloon made of goldbeater's skin, which is connected to the outside by a tube set in a cork. This balloon can be inflated or deflated simply by moving the elastic membrane. If the membrane is pulled down (fig. 37) the internal volume of the flask is increased by V while the internal pressure falls below that of the atmosphere. As a result a volume of air equal to V is displaced inwards and inflates the balloon. *This is the mechanism of inspiration.*

Conversely, if the membrane is relaxed (fig. 36) it recoils and the volume of the flask is reduced by the same volume V while the internal pressure rises. The air inside the balloon is driven out. *This is the mechanism of expiration.*

Thus **respiration depends upon the increase or decrease in the thoracic volume** (fig. 38). If initially the thorax is taken as a *truncated ovoid* with base ACBD, transverse diameter CD, anteroposterior diameter AB and vertical diameter SP, then the action of the inspiratory muscles, especially the diaphragm, increases all its diameters so that a greater ovoid A′C′B′D′ results with transverse diameter C′D′, anteroposterior diameter A′B′ and vertical diameter SP′. This situation differs from Funck's experiment in that *all the diameters of the container are increased* but the *similarities are quite striking* (fig. 39): the tube represents the trachea; the balloon represents the lungs; the elastic membrane represents the diaphragm. Two points need stressing:

on the one hand, the lungs fill the whole thoracic cavity and are connected to the thoracic wall by the *pleura* with its potential space. In fact its two layers are normally apposed and slide freely one on the other, thus ensuring *a tight mechanical link between the lungs and the thoracic wall*;

during inspiration the intrathoracic pressure falls and becomes negative not only relative to the outside but also *relative to the abdominal cavity*. As a result air enters the trachea and the lungs and *the venous return to the right atrium (RA) is speeded up*. Thus inspiration improves cardiac filling and, with the help of the lesser circulation, *brings venous blood into contact with the newly inspired air*. Thus inspiration **at once ensures air entry and pulmonary vascular perfusion**.

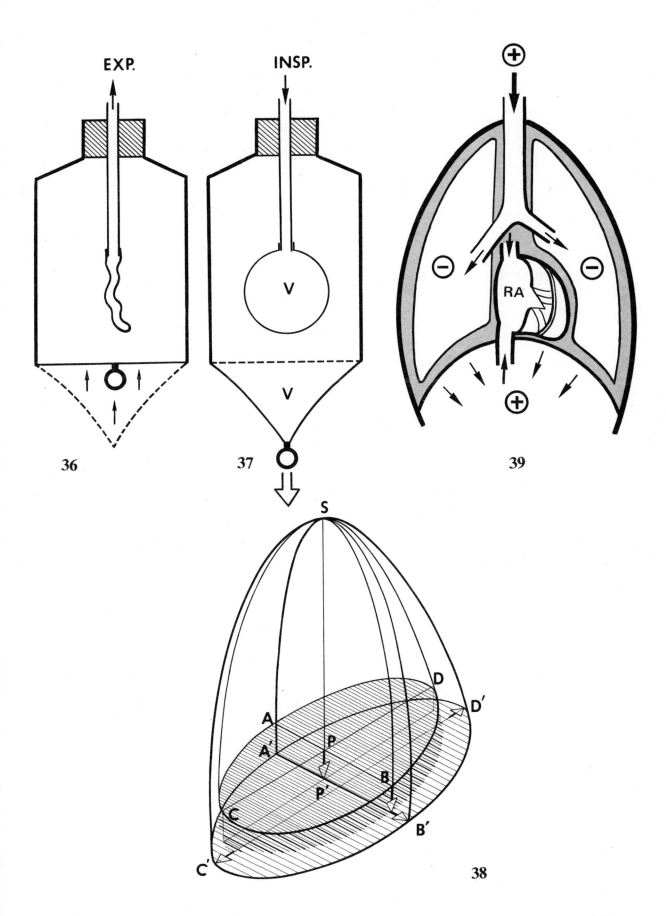

EXP.

INSP.

V

V

36

37

$\oplus$

$\ominus$ RA $\ominus$

$\oplus$

39

S

A
A'
P
B
P'
C
B'
C'
D
D'

38

153

RESPIRATORY VOLUMES

Respiratory or pulmonary volumes are simply the volumes of air displaced during the various phases and modes of respiration.

We have found it useful to represent these various volumes by the pleats of an accordion, as it makes for easy comparison.

During quiet respiration (fig. 40) the various respiratory volumes can be defined as follows:

the air displaced between normal inspiration and normal expiration is the **tidal volume**, i.e., 500 ml. This is shown as a grey band (2), with the oscillations of the spirogram;

if normal inspiration is prolonged into *forced inspiration*, the extra volume inhaled represents the **inspiratory reserve volume** (IRV), i.e., 1500 ml;

the sum of the inspiratory reserve volume and the tidal volume is the **inspiratory capacity** (IC), i.e., 2000 ml;

if a normal expiration is prolonged into forced expirtation to the maximum, the extra volume exhaled is the **expiratory reserve volume** (ERV), i.e., 1500 ml;

the sum of the inspiratory reserve volume, the tidal volume and the expiratory reserve volume is the **vital capacity** (VC), i.e., 3500 ml;

after a complete expiration some air is still present in the bronchi and lungs—the **residual volume** (RV), i.e., 500 ml;

the sum of the residual volume and the expiratory reserve volume is the **functional residual capacity** (FRC), i.e., 2000 ml;

finally the sum of the vital capacity and the residual volume is the **total capacity**, i.e., 4000 ml.

During exercise (fig. 4) the various volumes are distributed differently within the total lung capacity.

Only the *residual volume is unchanged* as it can never be expelled whatever the force of expiration.

On the other hand, as the respiratory rate increases, the *tidal volume* (TV) rises to a maximum but as the respiratory rate keeps increasing the tidal volume tends to fall slightly. The product of respiratory rate and tidal volume is **respiratory minute volume**, which therefore eventually reaches a maximum.

The *expiratory reserve volume increases markedly* indicating that the depth of rapid respiration during exercise approaches the maximum amplitude allowed by the thoracic cage.

As a result of the increase in tidal volume and expiratory reserve volume *the inspiratory reserve volume falls.*

RESPIRATORY VOLUMES AT REST

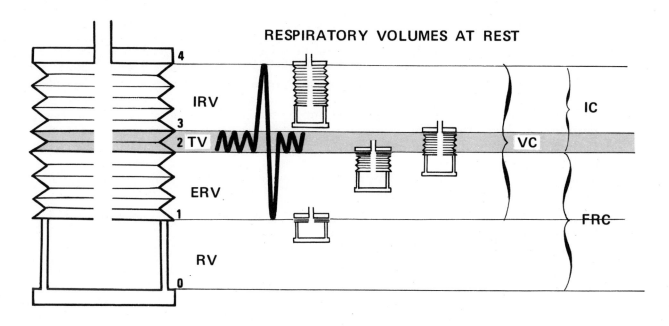

40

RESPIRATORY VOLUMES DURING EXERCISE

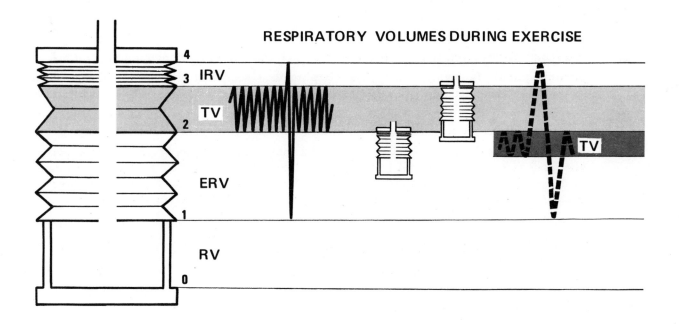

41

THE PATHOPHYSIOLOGY OF RESPIRATION

Many factors can interfere with respiratory efficiency.

Funck's experiment (fig. 42) can be modified as follows. If part of the flask wall is replaced by *another elastic membrane*, it follows that when the bottom membrane is pulled down, the second membrane is sucked in by a volume v, which *reduces* the inflating volume of the balloon to $V - v$. This occurs in man as the **flail chest**: a variable portion of the thoracic cage fails to follow the movements of the cage and is sucked in during inspiration leading to **paradoxical respiration**. This decreases respiratory efficiency leading to respiratory distress. If the pleura communicates with the outside through a wound, the underlying lung recoils inwards from its own elasticity and at every inspiration air enters the wound giving rise to a *traumatic pneumothorax*. This results in great respiratory distress and life is precariously maintained by the other lung provided it is healthy.

Fig. 43 shows the **various factors—mostly respiratory—that can interfere with normal blood-gas exchange**:

a pneumothorax (1), *where the pleural cavity fills up with air as a result of a pleuropulmonary fistula*, or *rupture of a bronchus or of an emphysematous bulla*. Here the pleura fails to pull on the lung;

a haemothorax, a hydrothorax or a pleural exudate (2), lying on the diaphragmatic surface. This leads to retraction of the lung with loss of function;

the flail chest (4);

atelectasis, secondary to bronchial obstruction. In the diagram the left upper lobe is atelectatic due to obstruction of the upper lobe bronchus;

inflammatory pleural thickening (6), due to an old pleurisy, a pyothorax or a haemothorax. The thick pleural shell hugs the lung tightly and prevents its expansion in inspiration;

acute gastric dilatation (7), which hinders downward movement of the diaphragm;

intestinal obstruction with distension (8), which pushes the diaphragm into the thorax;

phrenic paralysis (fig. 44): here the left phrenic is sectioned and the left dome of the diaphragm is paralysed and gives rise to *paradoxical movements*, i.e., instead of moving down it rises during inspiration.

Respiratory mechanics can also be significantly altered by the **position of the body**:

in the supine position (fig. 45), the abdominal organs push the diaphragm upwards *making inspiration more difficult*. The tidal volume is displaced upwards on the diagram at the expense of the inspiratory reserve volume. This occurs under anesthesia and can be aggravated by anaesthetics and muscle relaxants which reduce the efficiency of the respiratory muscles;

when one lies on one side (fig. 46), the diaphragm is pushed upwards far more on the lower side. The *lower lung is less efficient than the other* and, to make matters worse, *circulatory stasis* also supervenes. Anaesthetists particularly dread this position.

Respiratory mechanics also **vary with age and sex** (fig. 47). In women, respiration is *upper thoracic* with the maximum range of movement seen in the upper thorax, which shows an increase in its anteroposterior diameter. *In the child* it is *abdominal* and *in man* it is *mixed, i.e., upper and lower thoracic*.

In the aged (fig. 48) it is greatly altered by *accentuation of thoracic curvature* and *loss of tone of the abdominal muscles*. As the curvature of the upper thorax increases the upper ribs are approximated and their movements curtailed. Thus the upper lobe is poorly aerated and breathing becomes *lower thoracic or even abdominal*.

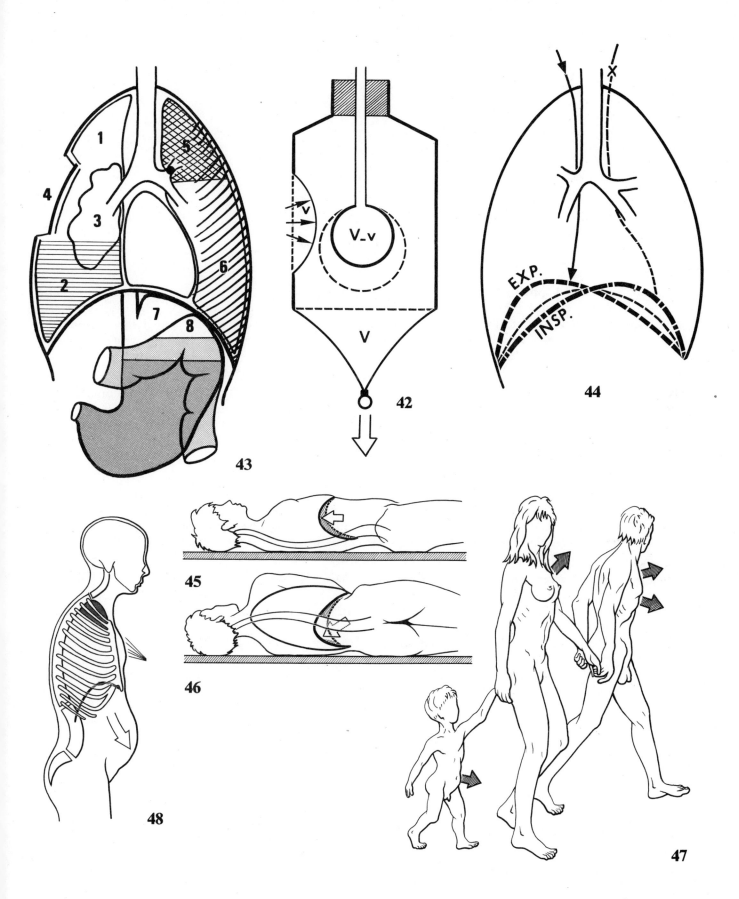

42

43

44

45

46

47

48

157

THE DEAD SPACE

The **dead space** is the *volume of air that does not participate in respiratory exchange*. In fig. 49 if the 'exhaust pipe' is widened at its tip by a container of volume DS, the dead space is increased. In fact, if only the tidal volume of 500 ml is being displaced and if the addition to the dead space has also a volume of 500 ml, then respiration only displaces air within the dead space and no exchange takes place.

The *case of the diver* is easier to understand (fig. 51). Let us assume that he is connected to the surface only by a tube for breathing. If the tube volume equals his tidal volume at any time, whatever his respiratory efforts, he will be unable to inhale fresh air and he will only breathe in the air polluted by his own expired air. Thus he will rapidly die of asphyxia, as occasionally happened in the early days of diving. This problem is solved by conveying fresh air through a tube and allowing the expired air to be expelled by a valve in the helmet.

The **anatomical dead space** (fig. 50) represents the *volume of the respiratory airways*, i.e., the upper passages (mouth and nose), the trachea, the bronchi and the bronchioles. This equals 150 ml, so that during normal respiration only 350 ml participates in alveolar blood gas exchange. To increase its efficiency, one can either mobilise the inspiratory or expiratory reserve or decrease the dead space, as with a **tracheostomy** (T). This connects the trachea directly to the outside and *cuts down the dead space by almost half*.

However, tracheostomy is not without risks as it *deprives the respiratory tree of its normal defences* and exposes it to severe infections. In the diagram the respiratory volumes are represented by the pleats of an accordion (fig. 52) and the tracheostomy by the two openings at the base of the tube.

There is another type of dead space (fig. 53)—**the physiological dead space** (DS'), corresponding to a segment of the pulmonary system where ventilation occurs but *perfusion is cut off*, e.g., as a result of a pulmonary embolus (PE). Ventilation is wasted and the anatomical dead space is increased.

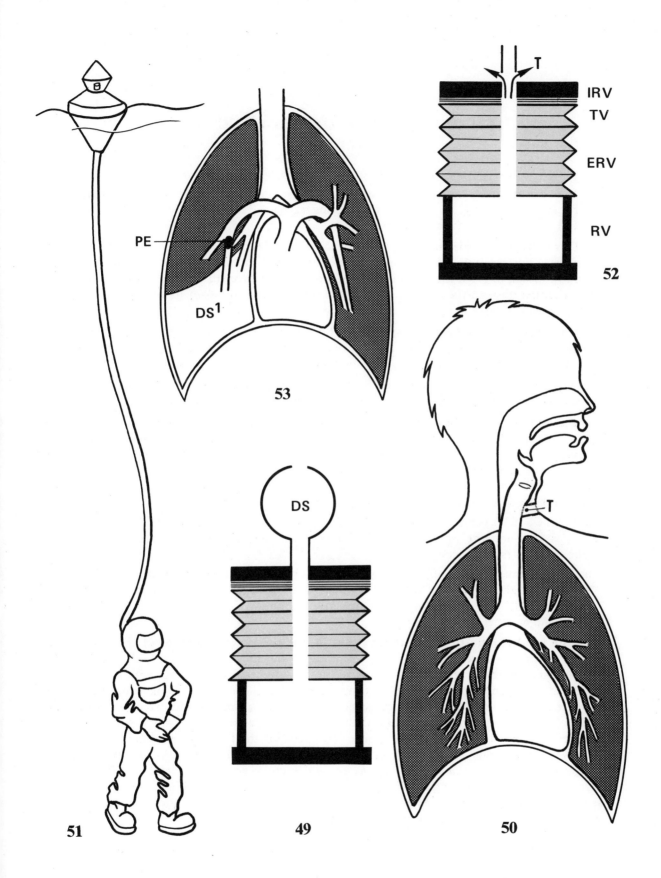

51

DS

49

PE

DS¹

53

IRV
TV
ERV
RV

T

52

T

50

COMPLIANCE OF THE THORACIC CAGE

Compliance is *directly related to the elastic components of the thorax and lungs.*

In **normal expiration** (fig. 54), the thorax and the lungs regain their position of equilibrium, which can be compared to the state of a spring at rest. Thus there is a *pressure equilibrium* between the alveoli and the atmosphere.

During **forced expiration** (fig. 53), the active muscles compress the elastic components of the thorax. For example, if the spring representing the thorax is compressed by a pressure equal to $+20$ cm of H_2O, the intrapulmonary pressure will exceed the atmospheric pressure and air will escape through the trachea, but the thorax will tend to regain its original position, like the spring which tends to regain its original position O.

Conversely **during forced inspiration** (fig. 56), the spring like the thorax is extended and a negative pressure of -20 cm of H_2O develops within the thorax. This results in air being sucked into the lungs but the elasticity of the thorax will again bring it back to its initial position.

These changes can be quantitated by using **compliance curves** which relate intrathoracic pressure changes and thoracic volume changes. Three such curves can be drawn:

the curve of relaxation pressure (T) in which zero pressure corresponds to the residual volume (V_R). This curve is the *resultant of the curve relating thoracic volume to the pressure acting on the lungs* (P) *and the curve relating thoracic volume to the pressure acting on the thoracic wall only* (S). It is remarkable that when the thorax is relaxed (i.e., corresponding to the residual volume) the pressures developed in the elastic components of the thoracic wall (P_S) and of the lungs (P_P) are *equal and opposite*;

at V_3, i.e., at 70 per cent of the total lung capacity, the pressure developed in the thoracic wall is zero and the pressure on the thorax is due entirely to the elasticity of the lungs (the two curves intersect at this point);

at V_2 (maximum expiration) the lungs have not entirely lost their elasticity as the curve P is still to the right of the zero line. This explains why, if air is allowed into the pleural cavities, the lungs can still recoil down to a minimum volume (V_P), when they lose all ability to recoil and to expel air.

The total elasticity of the thorax (fig. 58) can therefore be considered as a combination of two springs: a large spring (S) corresponding to the thoracic wall and a small spring (P) corresponding to the lungs. The thoracic wall functionally controls the lungs with the help of the pleura and this can be represented as a coupling of the two springs (B). This coupling however requires certain adjustments, i.e., compression of the large spring (S) and extension of the small spring (P) As these springs are coupled they can be represented as a single spring C which represents the total elasticity of the thorax (T). Hence if the link between lungs and thorax is destroyed each spring assumes its individual position of equilibrium (A). To come back to compliance, it *relates volume of air to the parietal pressure needed to displace it*. In the graph (fig. 57) the compliance is equal to *the slope of the curve in its midzone*. Therefore the compliance of the lungs themselves is greater than that of the thoracic wall, and the total compliance of the thorax is the algebraic sum of these two compliances.

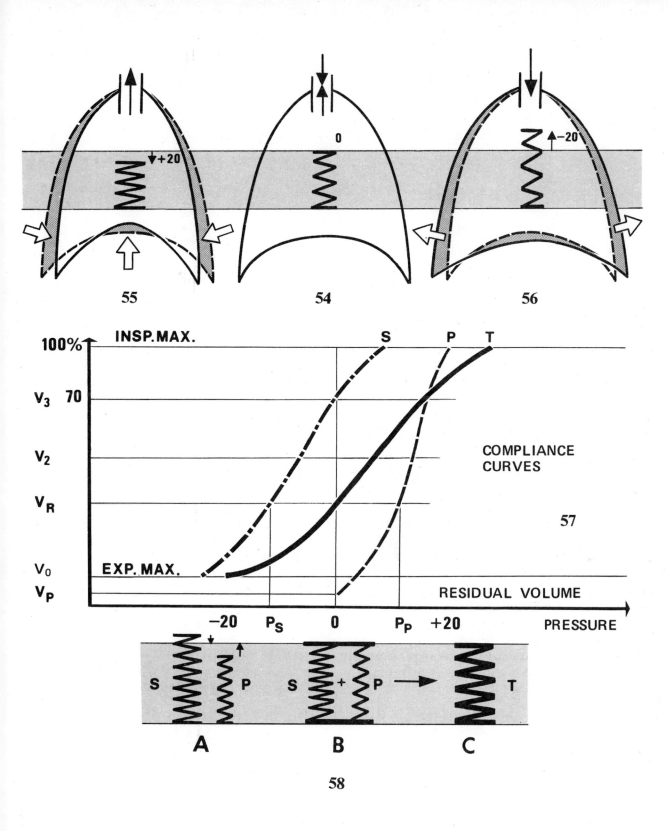

COMPLIANCE
CURVES

57

THE ELASTICITY OF THE COSTAL CARTILAGES

As already demonstrated (figs. 19 and 20), during inspiration the costal cartilages show an angular displacement due to axial rotation. This rotation also plays an important part in expiration. In inspiration the posterior ends of the ribs remain fixed to the vertebral column by the costovertebral joints (fig. 59) and, as the sternum is raised, the costal cartilages rotate about their long axes along the arrows t and t′. At the same time the **costochondral** (a) **and the sternochondral angles** are altered. (To make it easier to understand the sternum has been fixed and the vertebral column is considered movable.)

Diagrammatically, the costochondral and the sternochondral joints at each end of the cartilage can be viewed as *interlocking joints* (fig. 60).

The *medial end* (3) of the cartilage and the sternal edge (1) are tightly interlocked forming a solid angle completely filled by the cartilage. This allows some movement vertically but no rotation.

The *lateral end* of the cartilage (5) is shaped like a cone flattened anteroposteriorly and fits snugly into the anterior end of the rib which is correspondingly shaped. Here again slight lateral and vertical movements are possible but there is no rotation.

During inspiration, when the rib is lowered relative to the sternum, the costal cartilage twists on its own axis through an angle equal to t, and thus behaves like a **torsion rod**, which is used as a shock-absorber for cars. Thus, if a rod is twisted on its long axis, its elasticity stores the torsion energy which helps restore the rod to its original position when the force is removed. Likewise the energy of the inspiratory muscles is stored in the torsion bars of the costal cartilages during inspiration and, as these muscles stop acting, the *elasticity of these cartilages* brings the thorax back to its initial position. These cartilages are most flexible in youth and tend to ossify with age leading to a loss of thoracic flexibility and respiratory efficiency.

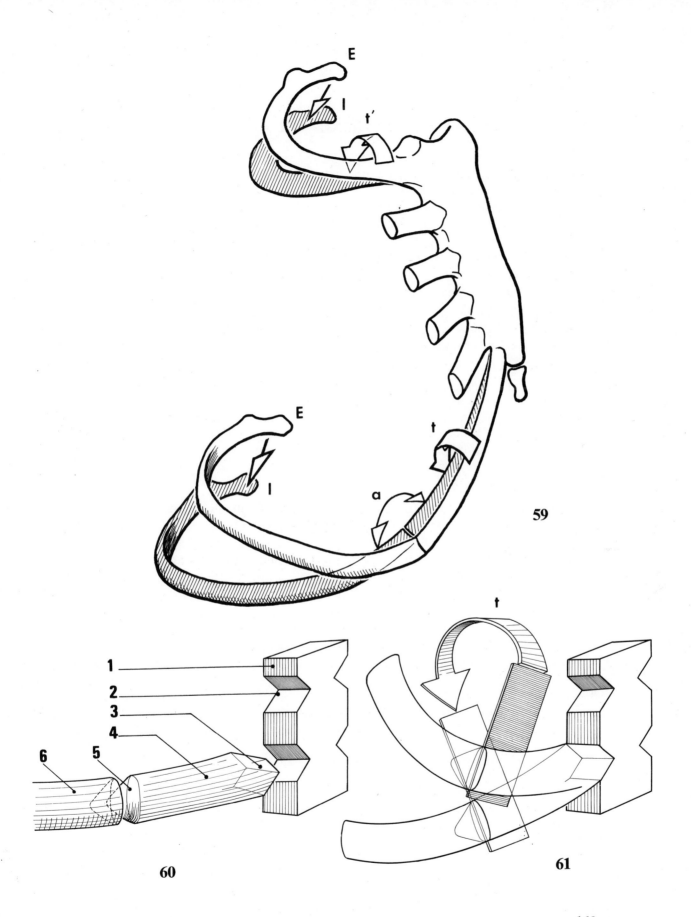

E

I

t'

E

t

I

a

59

1

2

3

4

6

5

t

60

61

THE MECHANISM OF COUGHING: THE CLOSURE OF THE GLOTTIS

As air enters the respiratory passages it is filtered, humidified and warmed by the nasopharynx. Theoretically it is free of suspended particles when it enters the trachea or the bronchi. However, if by accident foreign particles gain access to the bronchi an efficient mechanism is called into play—**coughing**. Likewise, coughing is involved in clearing the bronchial mucus secretions which trap fine particles and are constantly being wafted upwards by the cilia of the respiratory epithelium.

The **mechanism of coughing** can be analysed with the help of three diagrams which correspond to its three phases.

Phase I (fig. 62): *the inspiratory phase.* A deep breath is taken, moving into the lungs the bulk of the inspiratory reserve volume. The disadvantage of this deep inspiration is that it can carry down to the bronchioles any foreign matter lying below the glottis.

Phase II (fig. 63): *the pressure phase*, which involves the *closure of the glottis and the violent contraction of the intercostals and the accessory muscles of expiration, especially the abdominal muscles.* During this time there is a sharp rise in the intrathoracic pressure.

Phase III (fig. 64): *the expulsion phase.* While the accessory expiratory muscles are contracted the glottis opens suddenly releasing a violent current of air from the tracheobronchial tree. This carries along foreign particles and mucus secretions past the glottis towards the pharynx whence they are coughed up.

Therefore the efficiency of coughing depends on:

mobilisation of the abdominal muscles. Thus it is inefficient or absent in poliomyelitis with abdominal muscle paralysis and after abdominal operations when any contraction of these muscles is painful and avoided;

closure of the glottis requiring integrity of the larynx and its neural control.

Coughing is a **reflex act** set off by sensory receptors situated at the tracheal bifurcation and in the pleura. The afferent fibres of the arc are carried in the vagi, its centre is in the medulla and the efferent fibres go not only to the larynx but also to the intercostal and abdominal muscles. Its delicately balanced mechanism can be easily disturbed.

As already mentioned, closure of the glottis is essential for the cough reflex. The mechanism of closure of the glottis can be analysed diagrammatically as follows (figs. 65 and 66: seen from above; the numbers also apply to the figures on the next page). The glottis, seen from the pharynx, is a *triangular opening with its apex lying anteriorly* (fig. 65); its two edges are formed by the true vocal cords (15) stretching between the posterior aspect of the thyroid cartilage (3) and the anterior or vocal processes of the arytenoid cartilages (25), which are connected to the cricoid cartilage (7) [stippled grey in the diagram] by two joints whose *axes O and O' are approximately vertical. When the posterior crico-arytenoid muscles contract* (13) the arytenoid cartilages rotate about the joint axes O and O' and the vocal processes (25) are separated, opening the glottis. Conversely (fig. 66), when the *lateral crico-arytenoid muscles contract* (16) these cartilages rotate in the opposite direction and the vocal processes are approximated (25) bringing the vocal cords (15') into apposition and closing the glottis.

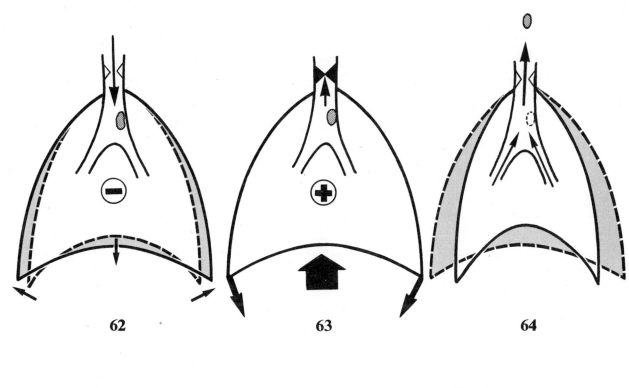

62   63   64

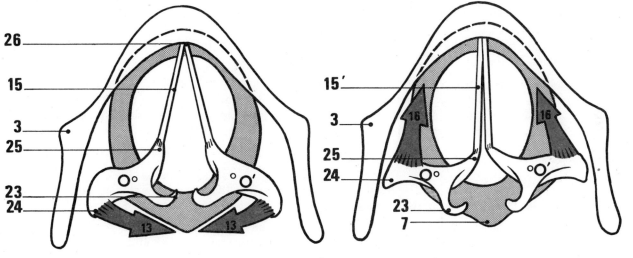

65   66

THE MUSCLES OF THE LARYNX AND THE PROTECTION
OF THE AIRWAYS DURING SWALLOWING

The larynx performs three important functions: the closure of the glottis *during coughing and the Valsalva manoeuvre, the protection of the airways during swallowing* and finally *speech*.

To understand these functions the **anatomy of the larynx must be reviewed**. A postero-lateral view (fig. 67) shows the cartilages joined to one another:

the *cricoid cartilage* (6) is ring-shaped (fig. 70) and has a posterior lamina (7) or signet-plate, which bears on either side two articular facets: the *inferior or thyroid facet* (22) related to the inferior horn of the thyroid cartilage; the *superior or arytenoid facet* (21) related to the arytenoid cartilage;

the *thyroid cartilage* has its posterior border visible (2); its anterior border is obscured by the oblique line (3), continuous with the superior horn which is attached to the hyoid bone by the thyrohyoid ligament. It consists of two laminae forming a solid angle anteriorly. To the inferior part of its posterior aspect (fig. 71) the true vocal cords are attached anteriorly (26);

lying on either side of the signet plate of the cricoid the *arytenoid cartilages* are roughly pyramidal in shape. They have three processes: the *superior process*, also called the *corniculate cartilage* (23); the *medial or vocal process* (25) giving attachment to the true vocal cord (15); *the lateral or muscular process* (24) giving insertion to the posterior crico-arytenoid muscle (13 and 14). Between the corniculate cartilage and the superior border of the signet plate of the cricoid runs a Y-shaped ligament, known as the cricocorniculate ligament, which bears a small cartilaginous nodule—the interarytenoid cartilage—at the junction of its inferior stem (12) with its two superior branches (10);

the *epiglottic* cartilage (1) is attached by its stalk to the posterior aspect of the solid angle of the thyroid laminae. Shaped like a leaf it is concave posteriorly and its long axis oblique superoinferiorly. Its two lateral edges are attached to the corniculate cartilage by two aryteno-epiglottic ligaments (9). Also seen (fig. 67) are the *right lateral cricoarytenoid muscle* (16), running between the muscular process of the arytenoid and the anterior border of the cricoid and the *right cricothyroid muscle* (17), running between the inferior border of the thyroid cartilage and the anterior border of the cricoid.

In fig. 68 the laryngeal inlet is marked by an arrow. It is bounded anteriorly and superiorly by the epiglottis, laterally by the aryepiglottic folds and the *aryepiglottic muscle* (19), inferiorly by the corniculate cartilages linked by the cricocorniculate ligaments (10) which are reinforced posteriorly by the transverse fibres of the *interarytenoid muscle* (18). The lateral walls of this inlet are also formed by the superficial fibres of the thyroarytenoid muscle (20). Here the inlet is shown open as in normal respiration.

During swallowing (fig. 69) the glottis is closed and *the epiglottis tilted inferiorly and posteriorly* towards the corniculate cartilages by the aryepiglottic (19) and thyroarytenoid muscles (20). Solid and liquid foods therefore slide on the anterosuperior surface of the epiglottis on their way down to the pharynx and the entrance to the oesophagus lying posterior to the cricoid.

The last two diagrams explain *how the glottis is closed* (fig. 70) and the vocal cords tensed during *speech* (fig. 71).

When seen from the front and the left side (fig. 70) the arytenoid cartilage (8) overlies the articular facet (21) of the signet plate of the cricoid (7).

This *crico-arytenoid* joint is synovial in type and its axis runs obliquely superoinferiorly, mediolaterally and posteroanteriorly. When the interarytenoid (18) and the posterior crico-arytenoid muscles (14) contract, the arytenoid swings laterally to a new position (shown in grey) and its vocal process (25) moves away from the midline. The vocal cords (15) therefore form a triangle with its apex in an anterior position. Conversely, when the lateral cricoarytenoid contracts, (16) the arytenoids swing medially, approximating their vocal process and the vocal cords (15').

During speech, the vocal cords are subjected to varying tensions, as seen in fig. 71. Taking the arytenoids as fixed, when the cricothyroid (17) contracts, the thyroid cartilage rotates about the axis of the cricothyroid joint (5) between the inferior horn and the side of the cricoid and its anterior part is lowered. The anterior attachment of the vocal cord moves from position 26 to 26', and the cord is lengthened; hence the cricothyroid *tenses the cord* (17'). This muscle, innervated by the recurrent laryngeal nerve, is the most important muscle of speech as it regulates the tension in the vocal cords and hence the pitch.

166

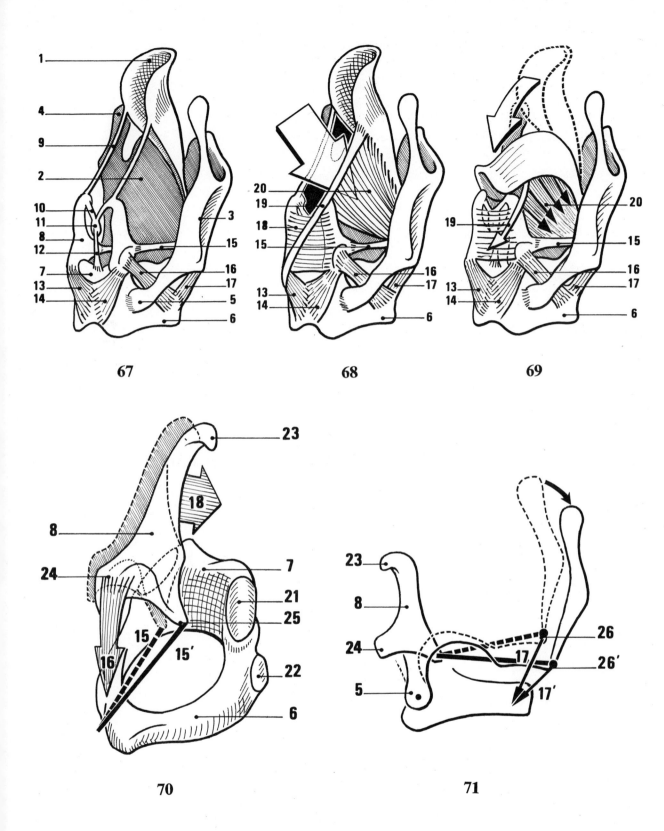

67

68

69

70

71

THE CERVICAL VERTEBRAL COLUMN

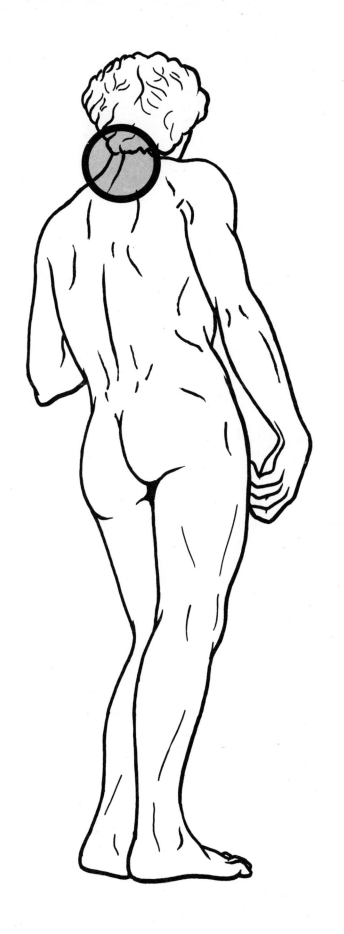

THE CERVICAL VERTEBRAL COLUMN TAKEN AS A WHOLE

Taken as a whole (fig. 1) the cervical column is made up of *two anatomically and functionally distinct segments*:

the superior or suboccipital segment (1), containing the first vertebra or *atlas* and the second vertebra or *axis*. These vertebrae are connected to each other and to the occiput by a complex chain of joints with three axes and three degrees of freedom;

the inferior segment (2) stretching from the inferior surface of the axis to the superior surface of T_1.

The cervical vertebrae are all alike, except for the atlas and the axis which differ from each other and from the remaining vertebrae. The joints of the inferior segment have only two types of movements: *flexion and extension*, and *lateral flexion with rotation*.

Functionally these two segments are complementary to allow pure movements of rotation, lateral flexion, flexion and extension of the head.

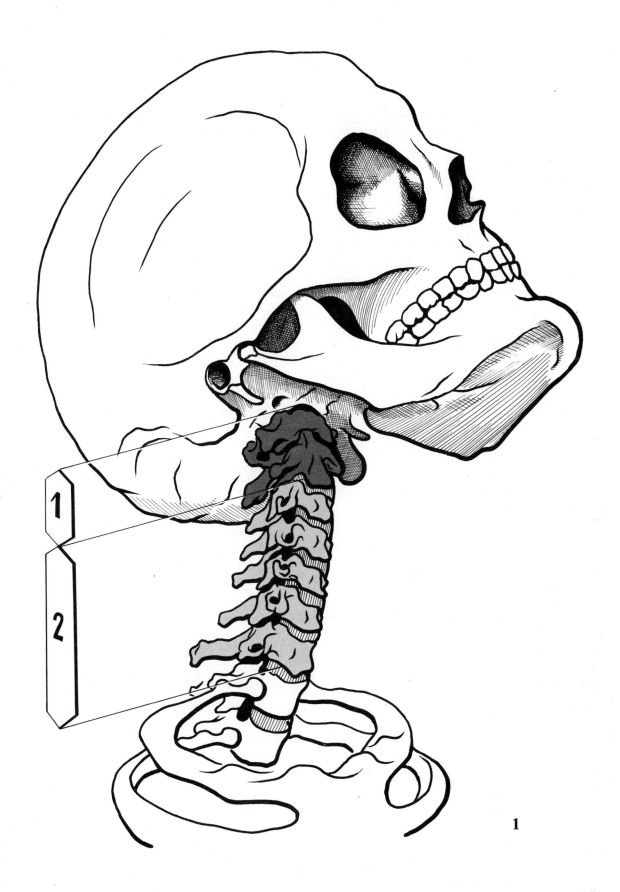

1

DIAGRAMMATIC REPRESENTATION OF THE STRUCTURE OF THE FIRST THREE CERVICAL VERTEBRAE

The atlas (fig. 2) is ring-shaped with its transverse diameter greater than its anteroposterior diameter. It has *two lateral masses* (1 and 1') oval in shape with their long axes running obliquely, anteriorly and medially; these in turn bear the biconcave *superior articular surface,* (2 and 2') facing superiorly and medially and meant for the occipital condyle, and *an inferior articular surface,* facing inferiorly and medially, convex anteroposteriorly and corresponding to the superior facet of the axis (12 and 12'). Its *anterior arch* (3) has on its posterior aspect a small cartilaginous oval-shaped *articular facet* for the odontoid process of the axis (11). The *posterior arch* (5) is initially flattened superoinferiorly but becomes thicker posteriorly to form the *posterior tubercle* on the midline (6). The *transverse processes* (7 and 7') have a foramen for the *vertebral artery* (8), which *deeply indents* the bone posterior to the lateral mass.

The superior surface (10) of the body (9) of the **axis** (fig. 3) carries centrally the *odontoid process* which acts as a pivot for the atlanto-axial joint, and laterally two articular facets (12 and 12'), which overhang the body laterally, face superiorly and laterally and are convex anteroposteriorly and flat transversely. The *posterior arch* (16) consists of *two narrow laminae* (15 and 15'), which are oblique posteriorly and medially. The *spinous process* (18) has two tubercles like every other cervical vertebra. The cartilage-lined *inferior articular processes* (17 and 17') are attached below the pedicle (16), face inferiorly and anteriorly and correspond to the superior articular processes of C₃ (24 and 24'). The *transverse processes* (13 and 13') have a vertical foramen (14) for the *vertebral artery.*

The **third cervical vertebra** (fig. 4) is similar to the last four cervical vertebrae and as such is a typical cervical vertebra. It has a vertebral body (19), like a paralleliped which is wider than it is high. Its superior surface, or *the superior plateau* (20), is raised laterally to form the *unciform processes* (22 and 22'), which face superiorly and medially and are connected to two flattened bony projections from the inferior surface of the axis. The anterior border of the plateau is also raised into a *ledge-like articular surface* (21), which faces superiorly and anteriorly and is connected to the posterior aspect of a bony prolongation of the overlying axis. The *inferior vertebral plateau* resembles the superior plateau and its anterior border shows a beak-like projection downwards.

The posterior arch bears: the *articular processes* (23 and 23'), which have a *superior articular facet* (24 and 24'), looking superiorly and posteriorly and corresponding to the inferior articular facet of the overlying vertebra (17), and an *inferior articular facet,* looking inferiorly and anteriorly and corresponding to the superior facet of the underlying vertebra. These articular processes are attached to the body by the *pedicles* (25), which receive the *transverse processes* (26), also attached to the body. The transverse processes which are *gutter-like,* contain a round *foramen* near the body for the passage of the vertebral artery and their extremities have an *anterior and a posterior tubercle.* The *two laminae* (27 and 27'), which are oblique inferiorly and laterally, meet in the midline to form the *spinous process* (28) with its *two tubercles.*

172

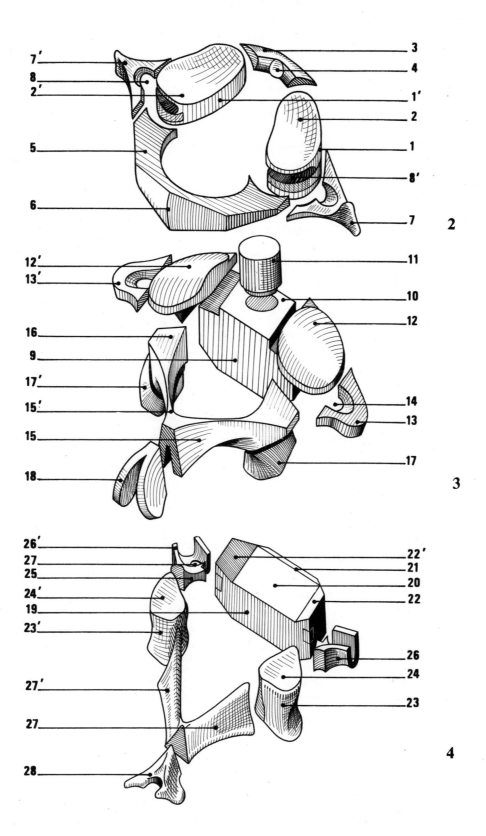

7′

8

2′

5

6

3

4

1′

2

1

8′

7

2

12′

13′

16

9

17′

15′

15

18

11

10

12

14

13

17

3

26′

27

25

24′

19

23′

27′

27

28

22′

21

20

22

26

24

23

4

173

THE ATLANTO-AXIAL JOINT

The mechanical link between the atlas and the axis is achieved by *three joints mechanically linked.*

A central joint, the **atlanto-odontoid joint** with the odontoid process serving as a pivot (see page 178).

Two lateral joints, the **atlanto-axial joints**, which are symmetrical and are formed by the inferior surface of the lateral masses of the atlas and the superior articular surfaces of the axis.

In fig. 5 (axis, seen in perspective) and in fig. 6 (axis, seen from the side) one can appreciate the shape and orientation of its oval superior articular facet (5), which is *oval* with its great axis lying anteroposteriorly, *convex anteroposteriorly* along a curve represented by xx′ and *straight transversely.* Therefore its surface can be considered as part of a cylinder (C) with axis (Z) running laterally and slightly inferiorly so that the articular facet looks superiorly and slightly laterally. The cylinder, whose surface corresponds to the articular facet (shown as transparent), contains the lateral portion of the axis with minimal encroachment on the transverse process.

One can also see the peculiar shape of the odontoid process which is roughly cylindrical but *is buckled posteriorly.* It bears anteriorly a *shield-like articular facet* (1), *which is slightly biconvex and corresponds to the facet of the anterior arch of the atlas*; and posteriorly a cartilage-lined *gutter* which is concave superoinferiorly and convex transversely and is related to the *transverse ligament.*

A parasagittal section (fig. 7) through the lateral masses of the atlas reveals the orientation and the curvatures of the various articular surfaces:

the curved interspace of the *atlanto-odontoid joint* with its odontoid articular facet (1) and the articular facet of the anterior arch of the atlas (2) (cut in the median sagittal plane) has a centre of curvature Q, lying posterior to the odontoid;

the *superior articular facet of the lateral masses of the atlas* (3) is concave anteroposteriorly and looks directly posteriorly. It is connected to the occipital condyles;

the *inferior articular facet of the lateral masses of the atlas* (4) is convex anteroposteriorly with a centre of curvature O and a relatively short radius of curvature;

the *superior articular facet of the axis* (5) is convex anteroposteriorly with centre of curvature P and a radius of curvature equal to that of the former. The two surfaces (4 and 5) therefore lie against each other like two wheels. (The star represents the centre of flexion and extension for the atlas on the axis; see page 174);

finally, the *inferior articular facet of the axis* (6) faces inferiorly and anteriorly; it is not quite flat and its gently curved surface has a long radius of curvature and a centre of curvature R. It corresponds to the superior articular facet of the articular processes of C_3.

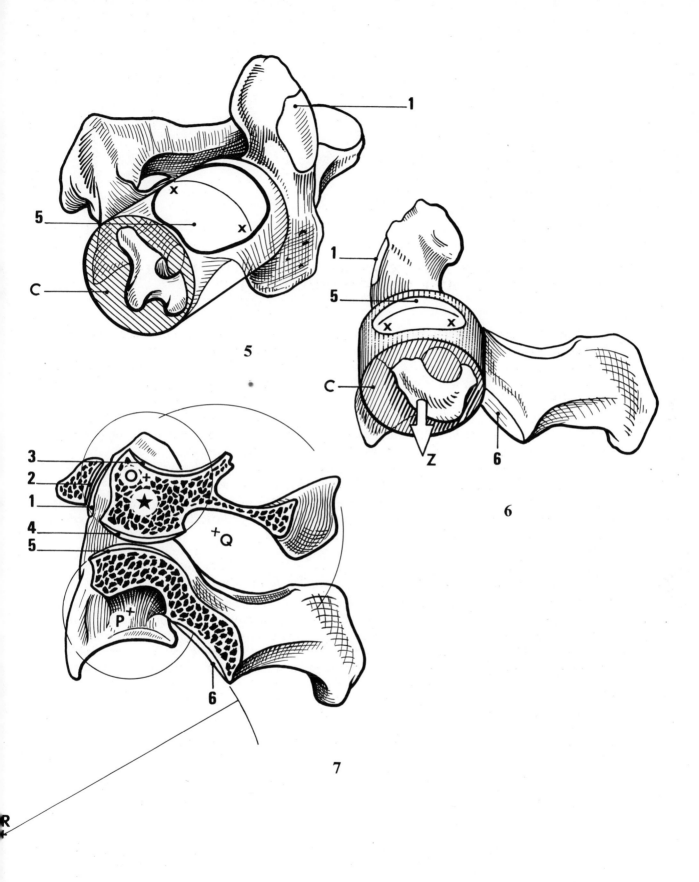

5

6

7

FLEXION AND EXTENSION IN THE ATLANTO-AXIAL AND ATLANTO-ODONTOID JOINTS

If one assumed that the lateral masses of the atlas rolled without sliding on the superior surfaces of the axis *during flexion* (fig. 8), the point of contact between these two convex surfaces would move forwards and the line joining the centre of curvature to the point of contact would move from PA to PA′; at the same time, the interspace of the atlanto-odontoid joint would open out superiorly.

Similarly *during extension* (fig. 9), the point of contact between these two surfaces would move backwards and the line PB would move to a new position PB′, and at the same time the interspace of the atlanto-odontoid joint would open out inferiorly.

In fact careful radiological studies *fail to show any opening out of this interspace* (fig. 10); this is due to the **transverse ligament** (T) which keeps the anterior arch of the atlas and the odontoid in close contact. The real centre, around which occur flexion and extension of the atlas over the axis, is neither the centre of curvature of the superior articular surface of the axis (P) nor that of the anterior facet of the odontoid (Q), but a third point (marked by a star) *lying more or less in the centre of the odontoid when seen from the side.* As a result during flexion and extension the inferior facet of the lateral masses of the atlas *rolls and slides* on the superior articular facet of the axis, just as the femoral condyldes on the tibial plateau.

It must be stressed that the presence of a *distortable structure,* i.e., the transverse ligament, allows some flexibility in the atlanto-odontoid joint. This ligament, fitting into the gutter on the posterior surface of the odontoid can *bend* upwards during extension and downwards during flexion. *This explains why the articular surface for the odontoid is not entirely bony.* The same applies to the annular ligament of the superior radio-ulnar joint, which is also a trochoid joint (see vol. I).

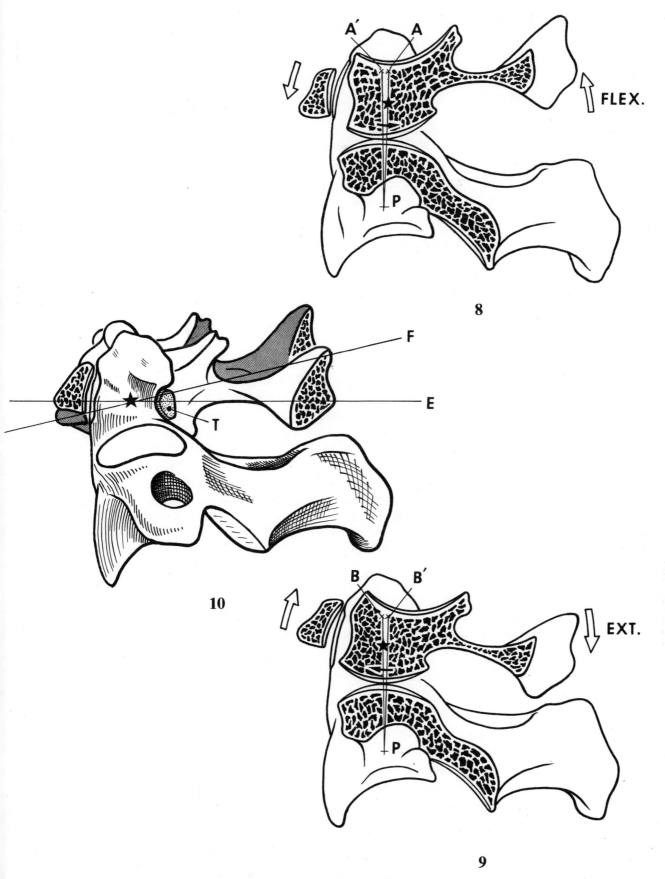

8

F

E

T

10

EXT.

B B'

P

9

177

ROTATION AT THE ATLANTO-AXIAL AND ATLANTO-ODONTOID JOINTS

When the atlanto-odontoid joint is viewed from above (fig. 11 and fig. 12 enlarged) it is easy to grasp its structure and to see how rotation takes place.

It is a *trochoid* consisting of two interlocked cylindrical surfaces:

a *solid cylinder*, the odontoid process (1), which is not strictly cylindrical, thus allowing the joint another degree of freedom, i.e., for flexion and extension. It has two articular facets, one anteriorly (4) and one posteriorly (11);

the cavity receiving this solid cylinder is an *empty cylinder* which completely surrounds the odontoid and consists anteriorly of the *anterior arch of the atlas* (2) and laterally of the *lateral masses of the atlas*. These masses bear on their medial surface a very distinct tubercle (7 and 7') to which is attached the powerful *transverse ligament* (6), running transversely posterior to the odontoid.

The odontoid is thus encased within an osteoligamentous ring and forms two types of joints with it:

anteriorly, a *synovial joint* (5) *with an articular cavity and a synovial capsule with two recesses*, one on the left (8) and the other on the right (9). The joint surfaces are the *anterior articular facet of the odontoid (4) and the posterior articular facet of the anterior arch of the atlas* (3);

posteriorly, a joint *without a capsule* and embedded in fibroadipose tissue (10), which fills the space between the osteoligamentous ring and the odontoid. The *articular surfaces are fibro-cartilaginous*, the one on the posterior surface of the odontoid (11) and the other on the anterior aspect of the transverse ligament (12).

During rotation, to the left for example (fig. 12), the odontoid (1) stays put while the osteoligamentous ring formed by the axis and the transverse ligament turns anticlockwise about an axis corresponding to the axis of the odontoid (white arrow), relaxing the articular capsule on the left (8) and stretching it on the right. At the same time *movement occurs in the right and left atlanto-axial joints* which are mechanically linked. During rotation from left to right (fig. 13) the left lateral mass of the atlas moves forward while the right lateral mass recedes and vice versa (fig. 14) during rotation from right to left.

But the superior surfaces of the axis are convex anteroposteriorly (fig. 16) and so the path taken by the lateral masses of the atlas is not straight in the horizontal plane but *convex* superiorly. Thus when the atlas rotates about its vertical axis W its lateral masses travel from x to x' and y to y'.

If one considers only the circle corresponding to the curvature of the inferior articular facet of the lateral masses of the atlas (fig. 15), it is clear that in the position of zero rotation the circle with centre O is at its highest on the superior surface of the axis. When the axis moves forwards this circle 'moves down' along the anterior border of the superior surface of the axis by a distance of 2 to 3 mm (e), while its centre moves down by half this distance (e/2). The same occurs when the axis moves backwards.

During rotation of the atlas on the axis, the atlas drops vertically by 2 to 3 mm so that its movement is really *spiral or helical*. The distance between the turns of this helix is very small and corresponding helices are obtained during rotation to the right or to the left.

178

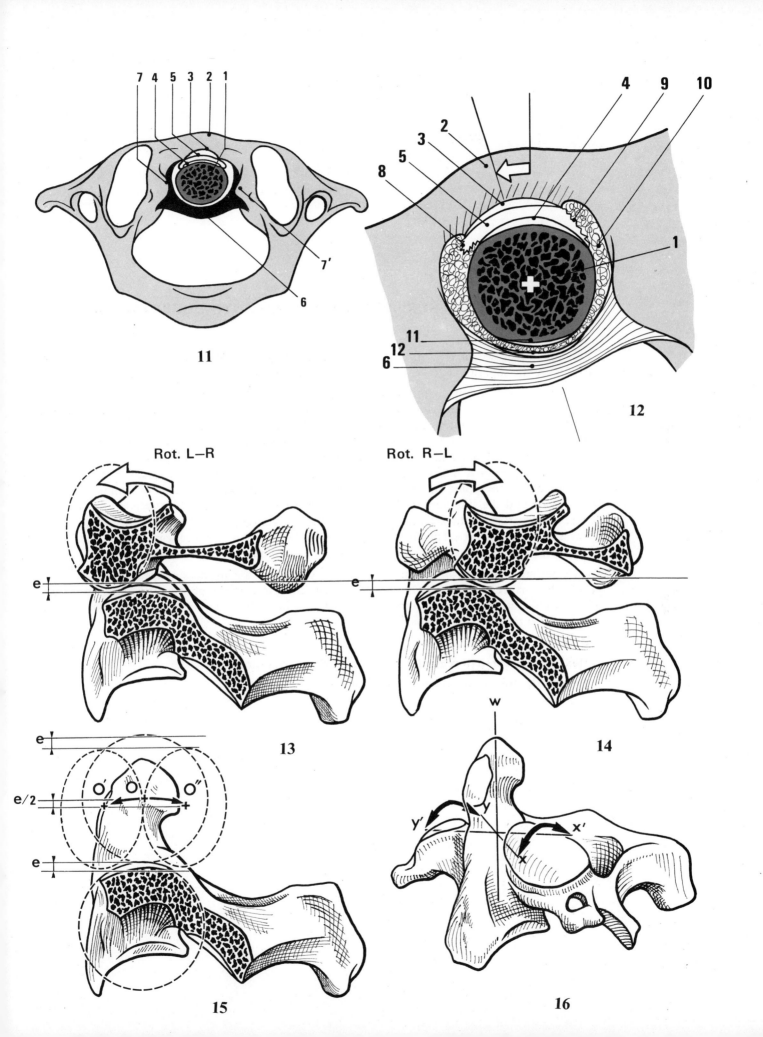

11

12

Rot. L–R

Rot. R–L

e

e

13

14

e

e/2

e

w

y'

y

x'

x

15

16

THE ARTICULAR SURFACES OF THE ATLANTO-OCCIPITAL JOINTS

There are in fact two such joints which are symmetrical and mechanically linked. Their articular surfaces are the superior articular facets of the lateral masses of the atlas and the occipital condyles.

In fig. 17 (atlas seen from above) the *articular facets of the atlas* are oval with their long axes running obliquely, anteriorly and medially and converging at a point N on the midline and slightly anterior to the anterior arch of the atlas. Occasionally they are waisted in the middle and may even be divided into two separate facets each. They are lined by cartilage and are concave in both directions with roughly similar curvatures. Therefore these surfaces can be considered as *part of the surface of a sphere* (fig. 19) with centre O located above the articular surfaces and vertically above the point Q, which is the point of intersection of the axis of symmetry of the lateral mass and the line joining the posterior border of the two articular facets. Q is also the centre of curvature of the articular surfaces in the horizontal plane. P is the centre of curvature of these facets in the vertical plane. Fig. 19 therefore shows that the sphere (considered transparent) rests exactly on the superior articular facets of the lateral masses of the atlas.

A posterior view of these joints (fig. 18) confirms that the surfaces of the occipital condyles also fit the surface of a sphere whose centre lies within the cranium above the foramen magnum. Therefore the atlanto-occipital joint is an *enarthrosis*, i.e., a joint with spherical articular surfaces (fig. 19) with *three degrees of freedom*:

axial rotation about a vertical axis QO;

flexion and extension about a transverse axis passing through O;

lateral flexion about an anteroposterior axis PO.

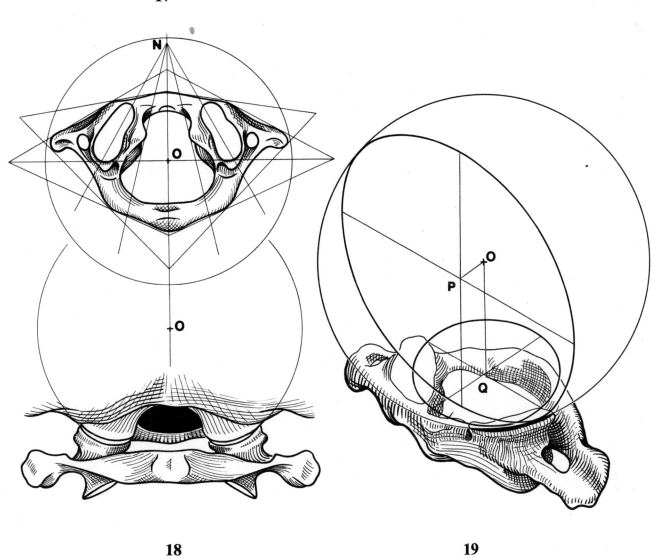

17

N

O

O

18

O

P

O

Q

19

ROTATION AT THE ATLANTO-OCCIPITAL JOINTS

When the occiput rotates on the atlas (fig. 20) its rotation is secondary to rotation of the atlas on the axis about a vertical axis passing through the centre of the odontoid. This rotation of the occiput is not simple as it actively stretches some ligaments, particularly the lateral *atlanto-occipital ligament* (L). The diagram, representing a frontal cut taken vertically through the occiput (A) and the lateral mass of the atlas (B), shows rotation to the left of the occiput on the atlas. This rotation is associated with an anterior displacement of the right occipital condyle on the right lateral mass of the atlas (arrow 1) but at the same time the lateral atlanto-occipital ligament (L) wraps itself around the odontoid and is stretched. *The tension developed in this ligament pulls the right occipital condyle to the left* (arrow 2).

Therefore rotation of the occiput to the left is associated at once with a linear displacement of 2 to 3 mm to the left and *lateral flexion to the right*.

Now, in classical dynamics a rotation associated with linear displacement is equivalent to another rotation of similar angle but with a different centre. Fig. 21 (seen from above) shows the atlas as light grey, the axis (viewed through the foramen magnum) as dark grey, the facets of the lateral masses of the atlas as horizontal stripes and the facets of the occipital condyles as oblique stripes (the condyles are considered transparent). During rotation to the left over an angle a about the centre of the odontoid O, the occiput is displaced to the left by 2 to 3 mm along the direction indicated by the vector V. It is now easy to appreciate that the **real centre of rotation** is P, lying slightly to the right of the midline and on the line joining the posterior border of the articular surfaces of the lateral masses of the atlas. Therefore the real centre of rotation moves between two extreme points, P for rotation to the left and P′ its mirror image for rotation to the right. It is interesting to note that this process brings into line the real axis of rotation at the atlanto-occipital joint and the anatomical axis of the brain stem.

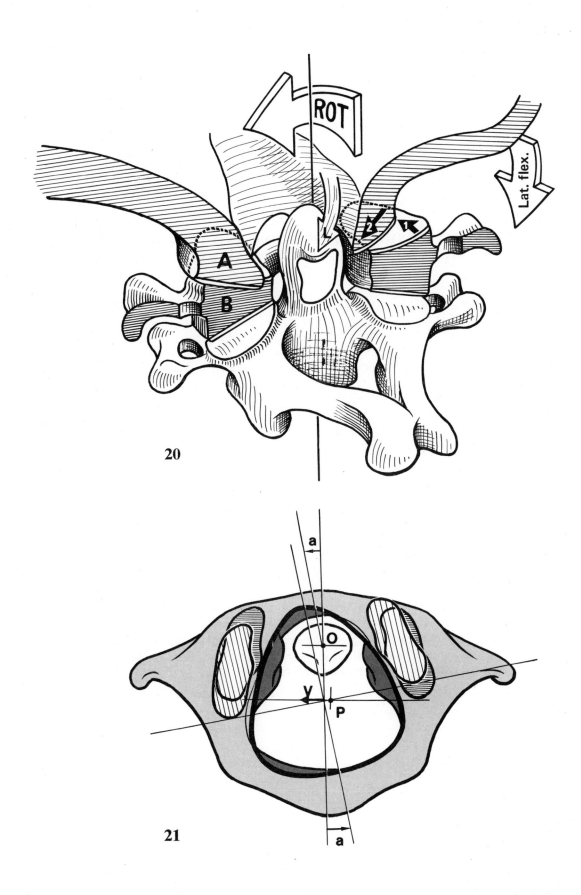

20

21

LATERAL FLEXION AND FLEXION AND EXTENSION
AT THE ATLANTO-OCCIPITAL JOINT

During lateral flexion (fig. 22), a frontal section taken vertically through the occiput, the atlas, the axis and C_3 shows that there is *no movement at the atlanto-axial joint*. Movement occurs only between the axis and C_3 and between the occiput and the atlas. Between *the occiput* and *the atlas* movement consists only of *the slipping* of the occipital condyles to the right during flexion to the left and vice versa in flexion to the right; there is a *small range of movement*. In the figure, showing flexion to the left, the left condyle and the odontoid are approximated without coming into contact because the movement is limited by the tension developed in the capsular ligament of the atlanto-occipital joint and especially in the right lateral odonto-occipital ligament. The total range of lateral flexion between the occiput and C_3 is 8°, with 5° between the axis and C_3 and 3° between the atlas and the occiput.

During flexion and extension of the occiput on the atlas the occipital condyles slide on the lateral masses of the atlas.

During flexion (fig. 23), the occipital condyles recede on the lateral masses of the atlas and, at the same time, the occipital bone moves away from the posterior arch of the atlas. As the latter movement is always associated with extension in the atlanto-axial joint the posterior arches of the atlas and axis become more widely separated. Flexion is limited by the tension developed in the articular capsules and the ligaments (the posterior atlanto-occipital membrane and the posterior cervical ligament).

During extension (fig. 24), the occipital condyles slide anteriorly on the lateral masses of the atlas. At the same time the occipital bone moves nearer to the posterior arch of the atlas and, as the atlanto-axial joint is also extended, the posterior arches of the atlas and axis are approximated. Extension is limited by the impact of these three bony pieces. During forced extension the posterior arch of the atlas can be caught as in a nutcracker and fractured.

The total range of flexion and extension is 15° at the atlanto-occipital joint.

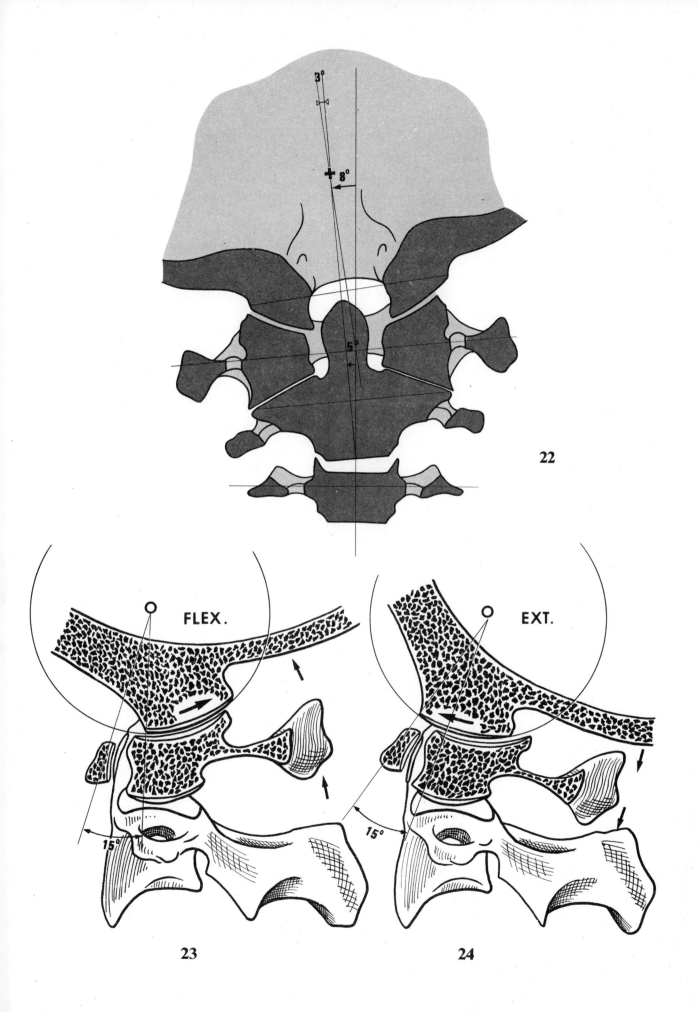

22

FLEX.   EXT.

15°   15°

23   24

THE SUBOCCIPITAL VERTEBRAL LIGAMENTS

(The numbers in the diagrams are common to figs. 25 to 33)

In figs. 25 to 33 the **bony structures** present are, from above downwards: the basi-occiput (a); the squama of the occiput (b); the anterior (e) and the posterior (f) arch of the atlas; the odontoid (g) continuous inferiorly with the body of the axis (k). On the odontoid are seen the anterior articular facet (h) facing the posterior articular facet (j) of the anterior arch of the atlas, and the posterior articular facet (i). Of the rest of the axis only the spinous process (n) and a section of its left lamina (o) are shown. Below the axis lies C$_3$ with its vertebral body (q), its spinous process (s) and a parasagittal section of its left lamina (r). Also seen in perspective are the cerebellar fossa above the foramen magnum, a segment of the right occipital condyle and the right half of the posterior arch of the atlas, the axis and C$_3$.

The **ligaments** in this region are numerous and strong:

the *cruciate ligament*, consisting of the *transverse ligament* (3), shown transected here and lying against the posterior articular facet of the odontoid (i); the *transverso-occipital ligament* (4) between the superior border of the transverse ligament and the basi-occiput; the *transverso-axial ligament* (5) between the inferior border of the transverse ligament and the posterior aspect of the body of the axis;

the *apical ligament of the odontoid process* (1), very short and thick, runs from the apex of the odontoid to the basi-occiput;

the *median occipito-axial ligament* (7), posterior to the cruciate ligament, runs from the basi-occiput to the body of the axis. It is continuous laterally with the *lateral occipito-axial ligament* (not shown here);

the *capsular ligament of the atlanto-occipital joint* (9);

the *posterior longitudinal ligament* (12), lying posterior to the median and lateral occipito-axial ligaments, runs from the gutter in the basi-occiput to the sacral canal;

the *anterior atlanto-occipital membrane* (16) is continuous inferiorly with the apical ligament of the odontoid. It is made up of an anterior (13) and a posterior (14) band and runs from the inferior aspect of the occiput to the anterior aspect of the anterior arch of the atlas;

the *anterior atlanto-axial ligament* (16) is continuous inferiorly with the anterior atlanto-occipital membrane. Thus the fibroadipose space, containing the atlanto-odontoid joint and its capsule (17), is bounded anteriorly by the odontoid and its apical ligament, and posteriorly by the anterior atlanto-occipital membrane and the atlanto-axial ligament;

the *anterior longitudinal ligament* (18) lies anterior to all these ligaments, arises from the inferior surface of the basi-occiput, bridges over the anterior arch of the atlas without any attachment and gains insertion into the anterior aspect of the body of the axis (18'). From there on it courses down to the sacrum on the anterior surfaces of the vertebral bodies, being attached to each intervertebral disc (18'') and the anterior border of each vertebral body.

The posterior arches are linked by the following ligaments:

the *posterior atlanto-occipital membrane* (19) runs from the posterior margin of the foramen magnum and the posterior arch of the atlas and is the homologue of the ligamentum flavum. It is pierced just posterior to the lateral masses of the atlas by the occipital artery and the first cervical nerve;

the *posterior atlanto-axial ligament* (21) runs between the posterior arches of the atlas and axis like a ligamentum flavum. It is pierced just posterior to the atlanto-axial joint by the second cervical nerve;

the *ligamentum nuchae* (22) connects all the cervical spines with one another, including those of the atlas and the axis;

the *posterior cervical ligament* (23), a thick fibrous band, is analogous to a supraspinous ligament. It is attached superiorly to the squama of the occiput in the midline and divides the muscles of the neck into a right and a left compartment;

the *capsular ligament* of the joint between the articular proces of the axis and C$_3$ (24) lies posterior to the intervertebral foramen which lodges the third cervical nerve;

a *ligamentum flavum* (29) connects the posterior arches of the axis and C$_3$.

186

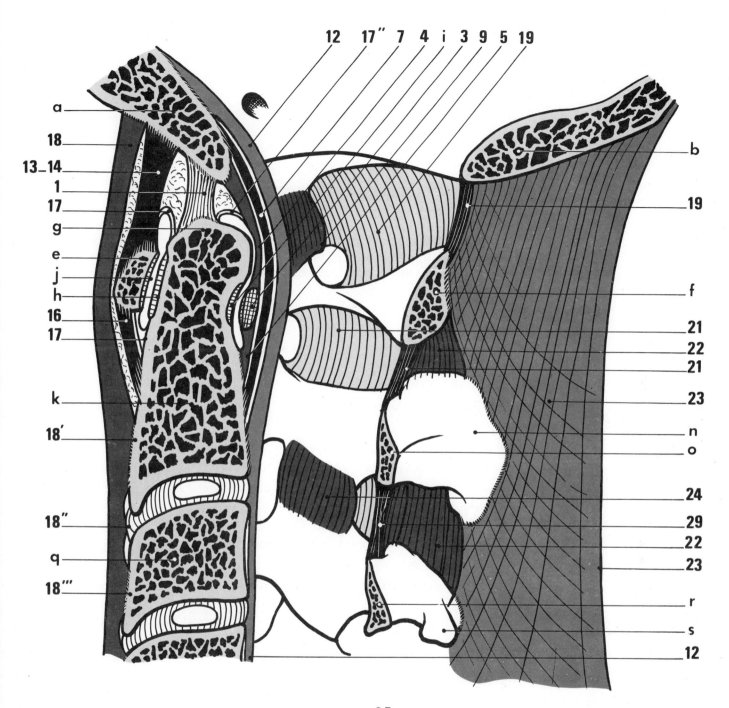

a

18

13 — 14

1

17

g

e

j

h

16

17

k

18'

18"

q

18'''

12   17"   7   4   i   3   9   5   19

b

19

f

21

22

21

23

n

o

24

29

22

23

r

s

12

25

THE SUBOCCIPITAL LIGAMENTS OF THE NECK

The arrangement of these ligaments is seen in fig. 26, which shows a frontal section of the vertebral column, taken vertically at the level of the posterior arches and viewed from the back after removal of these arches. The structures illustrated in fig. 25 are once more visible with the addition of the following:

the occipital condyles (c);

the lateral masses of the atlas (d);

the joints between the inferior articular facets of the lateral masses of the atlas (1) and the superior articular facets of the axis (m);

a section of the pedicle and of the articular process of the axis (t).

The following ligaments can be seen:

in the **deep plane** (fig. 27)—

the apical ligament of the odontoid (1);

the two alar ligaments of the odontoid (2);

the transverse ligament (3) running horizontally between the two lateral masses of the atlas;

the transverso-occipital ligament (4), which has been cut flush with the posterior margin of the transverse ligament and folded backwards;

the transverso-axial ligament (5), similarly cut and folded backwards.

in the **intermediate plane** (fig. 28)—

in the midline, *the crucial ligament* (6), made up of the transverse, the transverso-occpital and the transverso-axial ligaments;

laterally, *the capsular ligament of the occipito-axial joint* (9), reinforced laterally by the *lateral atlanto-occipital ligament* (10);

inferiorly, the *capsular ligament of the atlanto-axial joint* (11);

in the **superficial plane** (fig. 29)—

the median occipito-axial ligament (7) continuous on both sides with the *lateral occipito-axial ligaments* (8);

the posterior longitudinal ligament (12).

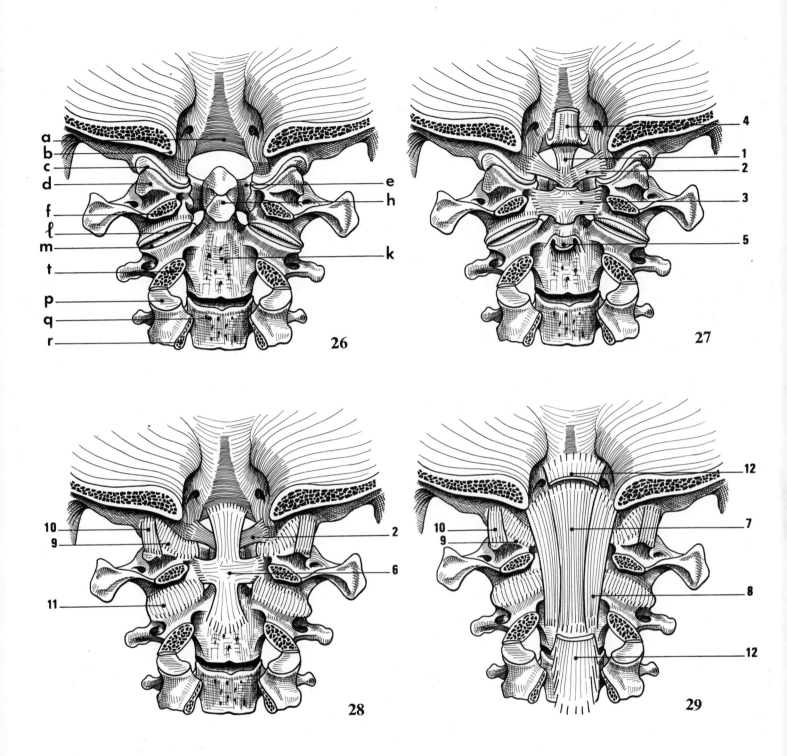

a
b
c
d
f
ℓ
m
t
p
q
r

e
h
k

26

4
1
2
3
5

27

10
9
11

2
6

28

10
9

12
7
8
12

29

THE SUBOCCIPITAL LIGAMENTS OF THE NECK (continued)

On the left side the diagrams show only the bony structures while on the right side the ligaments are also included.

Fig. 30 (viewed from in front) shows all the structures already described.

In fig. 31 the **anterior ligaments** are seen:

the *anterior atlanto-occipital membrane* with its deep layer (13) and its superficial layer (14), which overlies the *capsule of the atlanto-occipital* joint (9);

the *anterolateral atlanto-occipital ligament* (15), lying anterior to the former and running obliquely from the basi-occiput to the transverse process of the atlas;

the *anterior atlanto-axial ligament* (16), continuous laterally with the *capsular ligament of the atlanto-axial joint* (11);

the *anterior longitudinal ligament* (18) (only the left half is shown);

the *capsular ligament of the joint between the axis and* C_3 (23).

Fig. 32 (viewed from behind) shows the posterior arches of the atlas, axis and C_3, the vertebral canal and the foramen magnum between the occiput and the axis.

Fig. 33 (viewed from behind) shows on the right the ligaments covering the anterior aspect of the vertebral canal (also shown in fig. 29):

the *occipito-axial ligaments, median* (7) *and lateral* (8);

the *capsular ligament of the occipito-axial joint* (9) strengthened by the *lateral atlanto-occipital ligament* (10).

Also seen is the **vertebral artery** as it runs upwards through the foramina in the transverse processes and bends postero-medially to skirt the posterior border of the lateral mass of the atlas (25).

On the left side of fig. 33 the **posterior ligaments** are seen:

the *posterior atlanto-occipital ligament* (19), continuous with the *lateral atlanto-occipital ligament* (20) running between the squama of the occiput and the transverse process of the atlas;

the *posterior atlanto-axial ligament* (21);

the *ligamentum nuchae* (22), strengthened by the *posterior cervical ligament*, shown here only on the left side;

the capsular ligament of the joint between the axis and C_3 (24).

Also seen are the *first cervical nerve* (26) as it emerges through the foramen for the vertebral artery and the *second cervical nerve* (27), whose posterior ramus gives off the *greater occipital nerve*.

The posterior ramus of the third cervical nerve (28) is erroneously shown in the diagram, since it really emerges through the intervertebral foramen, i.e., *anterior* to the joint between the axis and C_3 (24).

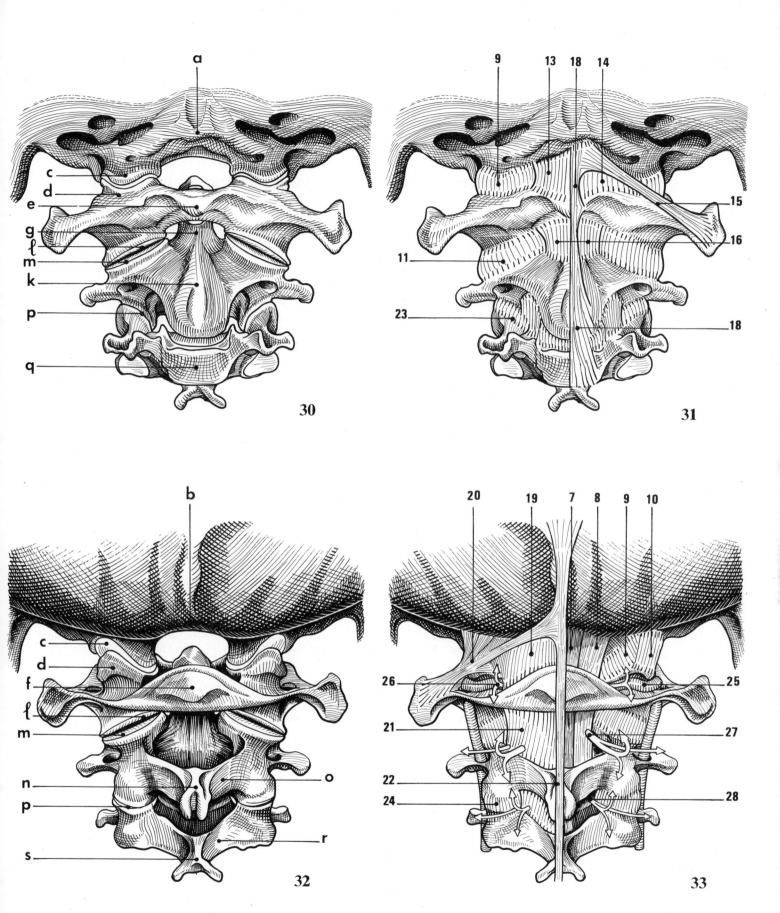

30

31

32

33

191

THE STRUCTURE OF A TYPICAL CERVICAL VERTEBRA

Fig. 34 shows a postero-superior view of an intact cervical vertebra and fig. 36 shows the same with its constituents 'exploded'. One can see the following:

the **vertebral body** (1) with its superior plateau (2) raised on either side by two buttresses, flat transversely—the *unciform processes* (3 and 3'), which harbour the corresponding articular facets on the inferior plateau of the vertebra. Also seen are the *ledge* (4) on the anterior margin of the superior plateau and the *beak-like prolongation* (5) of the anterior surface of the inferior plateau. As a whole the superior plateau is concave transversely and convex antero-posteriorly, resembling a saddle. It allows flexion and extension but lateral flexion is limited by the unciform processes which thus 'guide' the anteroposterior movements during flexion and extension.

On the posterior aspect of the lateral surface of the body are attached *the pedicles* (6 and 6') as they give origin to the **posterior arch** and the *anterior root of the transverse process* (7 and 7'). The transverse processes of the cervical vertebrae are peculiar in their orientation and structure. They are hollowed into a gutter anteroposteriorly and they point anterolaterally, forming an angle of 60° with the sagittal plane. They slope gently downwards at an angle of 15° with the vertical. The posteromedial end of the gutter lines the *intervertebral foramen* and its anterolateral end is bifid with *two tubercles*, anterior and posterior, which give attachment to the scalene muscles. Its medial portion is perforated by the foramen transversarium which lodges the vertebral artery. The cervical nerve, leaving the vertebral canal through the intervertebral foramen, thus crosses the vertebral artery at right angles, courses across the gutter of the transverse process and emerges between the two tubercles.

As the medial end of the transverse process is perforated it appears to arise by two roots, one attached directly to the vertebral body and the other to the articular process.

The **articular processes** (9 and 9') lie posterior and lateral to the vertebral body, to which they are connected by the pedicles (6 and 6'). They bear the *articular facets*; only the superior facets (10 and 10') are shown here and they correspond to the inferior facets of the overlying vertebra.

The posterior arch is completed by the *laminae* (11 and 11'), which meet in the midline to form the bifid *spinous process* (12).

The posterior arch is therefore made up in order by the pedicles, the articular processes, the laminae and the spinous process. The intervertebral foramen is bounded inferiorly by the pedicle, medially by the vertebral body and the unciform process and laterally by the articular process.

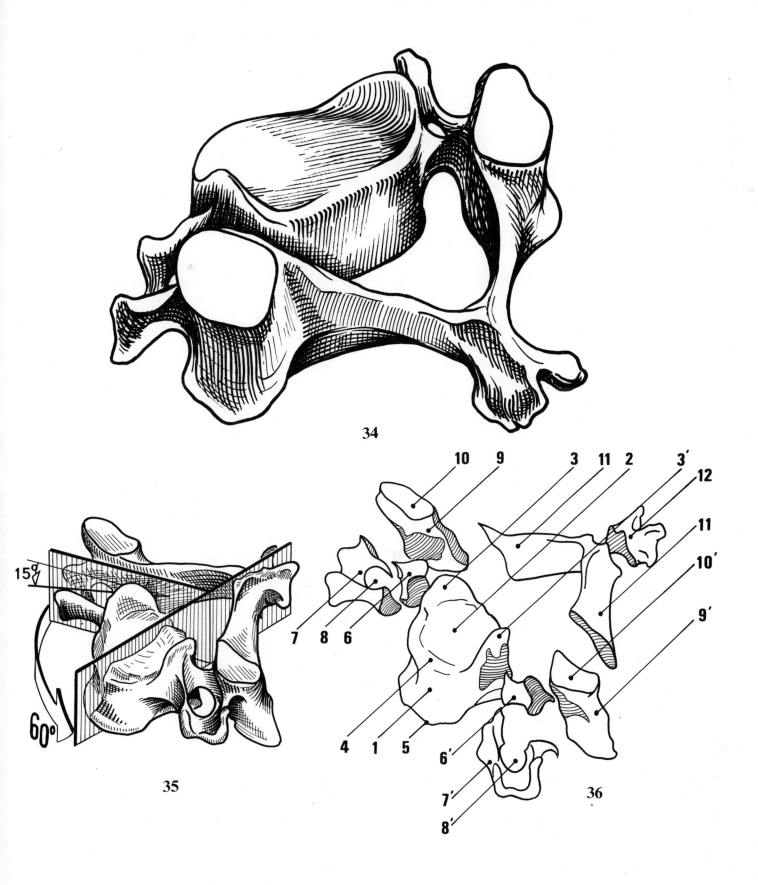

34

35

15°

60°

36

10 9 3 11 2 3′

12

11

10′

9′

7 8 6

4 1 5

6′

7′

8′

193

THE LIGAMENTS OF THE LOWER CERVICAL VERTEBRAL COLUMN

The special ligaments of the suboccipital region have already been illustrated and some of them extend down to the lower cervical region.

The lower cervical intervertebral ligaments can be seen in detail in fig. 37 (seen in perspective) which shows a vertebra cut sagitally with its superior plateau (a) and its raised unciform process (b), and an intervertebral disc with its annulus fibrosus (1) and its nucleus pulposus (2).

The *anterior longitudinal ligament* (3) and the *posterior longitudinal ligament* (4) lie respectively anterior and posterior to the vertebral body. On each side the unco-vertebral joints are bounded by a *capsule* (5).

The *joints between the articular processes* have one articular facet illustrated as (d) and their capsules are shown intact (6) and opened (6'). Between the laminae on both sides run the ligamenta flava (7), one of which has been sectioned (7').

The spinous processes (j) are interconnected by the *interspinous ligaments* (8), continuous posteriorly with a supraspinous ligament which is well defined in the suboccipital region as the *posterior cervical ligament* (9) and gives attachment to the trapezius and splenius muscles.

The transverse processes with their anterior (e) and posterior (f) tubercles are interconnected by *intertransverse ligaments* (10).

Also seen are the *foramen transversarium* (g) and the *intervertebral* foramen (i) bounded superiorly by the vertebral pedicle (h), posteriorly and laterally by the articular processes and their joint, and anteriorly and medially by the vertebral body, the intervertebral disc (1) and the unciform process (b).

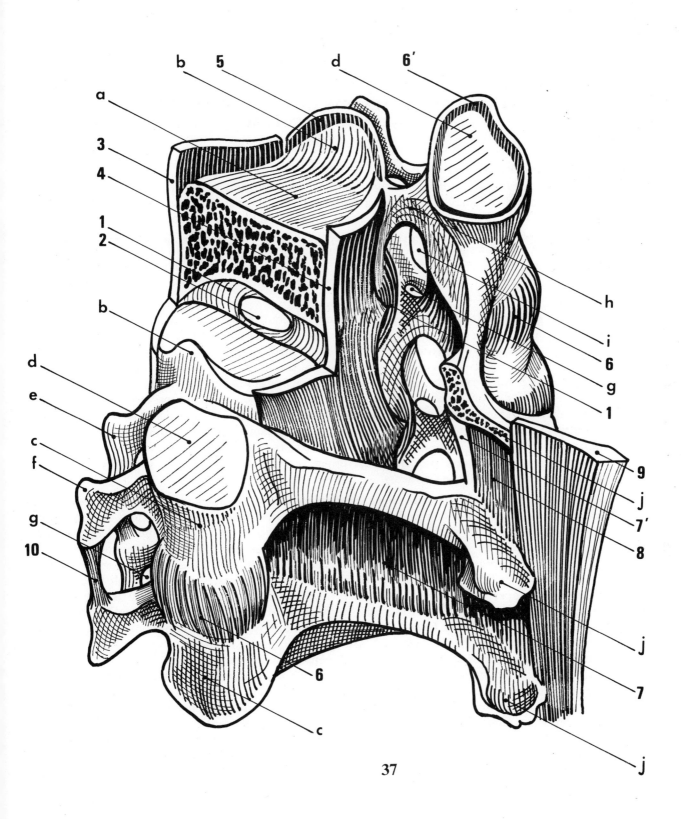

FLEXION AND EXTENSION OF THE LOWER CERVICAL VERTEBRAL COLUMN

In the neutral position, the vertebral bodies (fig. 38: seen from the side) are connected by an intervertebral disc, which is in the position of equilibrium with the fibres of the annulus uniformly stretched. They (fig. 39) are also connected by their articular processes whose articular surfaces are oblique inferiorly and posteriorly. At this level of the vertebral column these facets are slightly concave anteriorly in the parasagittal plane and their centre of curvature (marked by the cross) lies a long way inferiorly and anteriorly. As a result of the cervical lordosis, the centres of curvature of the articular surfaces of these processes are set farther apart than the planes of the articular surfaces themselves. On page 200 the significance of the convergence of these axes will be discussed.

During extension (fig. 40), the overlying vertebral body *tilts and slides posteriorly*. The intervertebral space is compressed posteriorly, the nucleus pulposus is driven slightly *anteriorly* and the anterior fibres of the annulus fibrosus are stretched. As this posterior sliding of the vertebral body does not occur about the centre of curvature of the articular facets of the articular processes, the interspace of the joints between these processes (fig. 41) is *widened anteriorly*. The superior articular facet not only slides inferiorly and posteriorly on the inferior facet but also tilts posteriorly with the formation of an angle x′ equal to the angle of extension x and to the angle x″ between the normals to the two articular facets. Extension is limited by the *tension developed in the anterior longitudinal ligament* and by the impact of the superior articular process of the lower vertebra on the transverse process of the upper vertebra and especially by the *impact of the posterior arches* through the ligaments.

During flexion (fig. 42), the upper vertebral body *tilts and slides anteriorly*, compressing the intervertebral space anteriorly and driving the nucleus posteriorly and stretching the posterior fibres of the annulus. This tilting of the upper vertebra is helped by the anterior ledge on the superior plateau of the lower vertebra which allows the beak-like projection of the lower plateau of the upper vertebra to move past. Just as with extension, flexion of the vertebra does not occur about the centre of curvature of the facets of the articular processes and as a result the inferior facet of the upper vertebra *moves superiorly and anteriorly* and the interspace is opened out posteriorly by an angle y′ which is equal to the angle of extension y and the angle y″ between the normals to two articular facets. Flexion is not limited by bony impact but only by the tension developed in the posterior longitudinal ligament, the capsular ligament of the joint between the articular processes, the ligamenta flava, the ligamentum nuchae and the posterior cervical ligament. During car accidents, with impact in front or from behind, the cervical vertebral column is strongly extended and then flexed. This produces the whiplash injury related to *stretching or even tearing of these various ligaments* and, in extreme cases, *to anterior dislocation of these joints*. The inferior articular facets of the upper vertebra become hooked on the antero-superior margins of the articular facet of the lower vertebra. This type of dislocation is difficult to reduce and endangers the medulla oblongata and the cervical cord with the risk of death, quadriplegia or paraplegia.

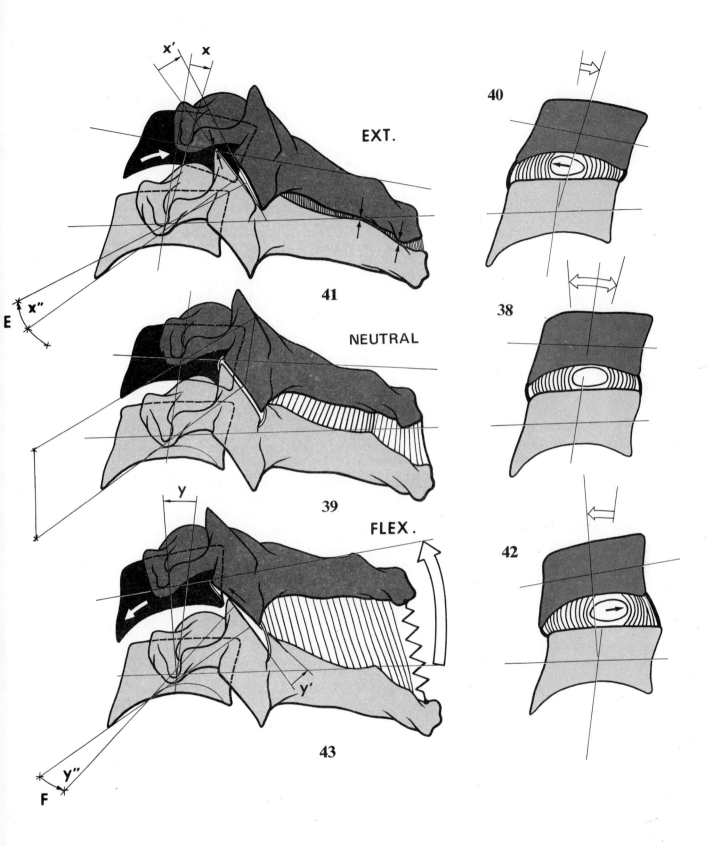

EXT.

41

NEUTRAL

39

FLEX.

43

40

38

42

197

MOVEMENTS AT THE UNCO-VERTEBRAL JOINTS

So far we have considered only movements at the joints between the articular processes and the intervertebral discs but in the cervical vertebral column movements also occur at two small additional joints—the **unco-vertebral joints (joints of Luschka).** A frontal section (fig. 44) shows the two vertebral plateaus, the disc with its nucleus and annulus, but the disc does not reach the lateral margins of the vertebra. In fact, the superior plateau is raised laterally by two buttresses lying in a sagittal plane. These *unciform processes* have their cartilage-lined articular surfaces facing medially and superiorly and corresponding to the cartilage-lined *semilunar facets* of the inferior plateau of the upper vertebra, the latter facets pointing inferiorly and laterally. These small joints are enclosed within a *capsule* continuous medially with the intervertebral disc.

During flexion and extension, when the body of the upper vertebra slides anteriorly or posteriorly, the articular facets of the unco-vertebral joints also slide relative to each other. Thus these unciform processes 'guide' the vertebral body into this anteroposterior movement.

During lateral flexion (fig. 45) the interspaces of the unco-vertebral joints *open out* by an angle a′ or a″ equal to the angle of lateral flexion a, and to the angle formed between the two horizontal lines nn′ and nm′ joining the transverse processes. Also shown are the contralateral displacement of the nucleus and the stretching of the capsule of the contralateral unco-vertebral joint.

In reality the movements at the unco-vertebral joints are *far more complex*. We shall see later that pure lateral flexion does not occur but is *always associated with rotation and extension*. Therefore during these movements the interspace of the unco-vertebral joint gapes not only *superiorly or inferiorly but also anteriorly as the upper vertebra moves backwards*. The diagrams (figs. 46A and B: seen in perspective), where the vertebrae are extremely simplified, are meant to demonstrate these movements more clearly. It would be a good idea to come back to these diagrams after grasping the mechanism of combined lateral flexion and rotation.

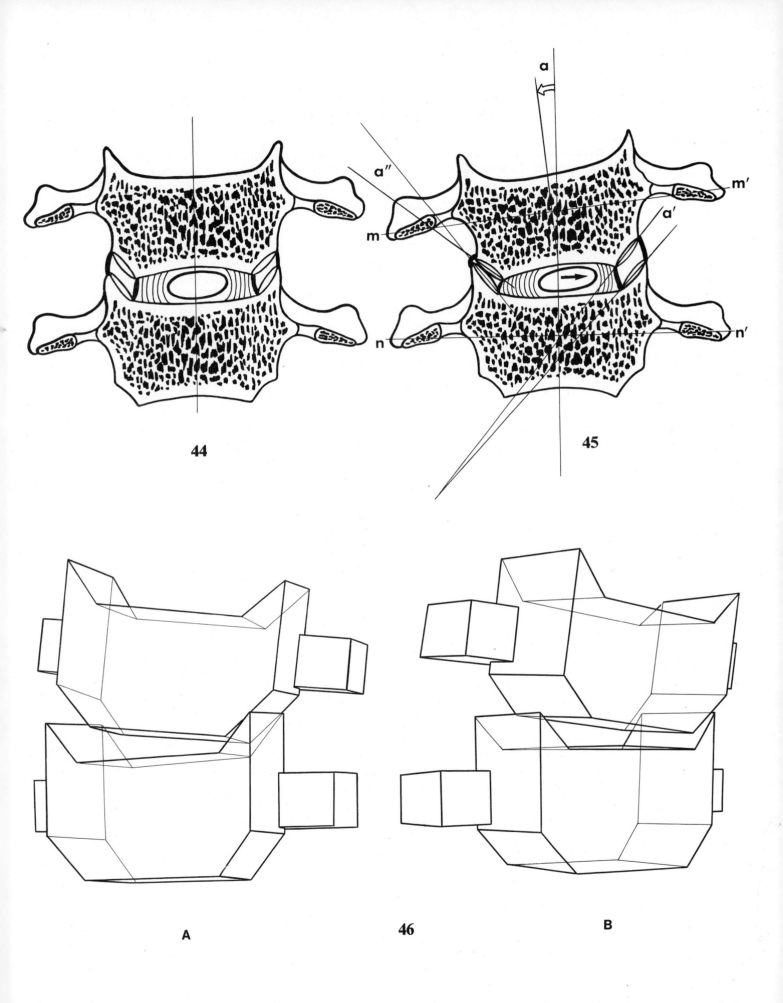

44

45

A   **46**   **B**

THE ORIENTATION OF THE ARTICULAR FACETS:
THE COMPOSITE AXIS OF COMBINED ROTATION AND LATERAL FLEXION

Lateral flexion and rotation in the lower cervical vertebral column are *governed by the orientation of the facets* of the articular processes, which prevents pure rotation or pure lateral flexion.

If one considers a vertebra in the middle of the cervical column, *e.g.*, C_5 (fig. 47), its superior articular facets are *flat and lie in the same plane P, oblique inferiorly and posteriorly*. Thus any sliding of C can only be of two types:

combined, with both facets moving *superiorly during flexion* or *inferiorly during extension*;

differential or relative, with the left facet moving superiorly and anteriorly (arrow a) while the right facet moves inferiorly and posteriorly (arrow b). This relative sliding in the plane P is therefore tantamount to *rotation* about an *axis A perpendicular to plane P* and lying in the sagittal plane and so on the line perpendicular to that joining the centres of the articular facets of C_5. Therefore the movement involved is a **combination of rotation and lateral flexion** depending on the obliquity of the axis A.

Horizontal sections taken at various levels of the joints between the articular processes (fig. 48) show that the superior and inferior surfaces of these facets are not strictly flat but are slightly convex posteriorly between C_6 and C_7 (fig. 48A) or slightly concave posteriorly between C_3 and C_4 (B). This observation in no way contradicts what has already been described, since one can replace the plane P (fig. 47) by a *spherical surface of large radius with centre lying on the axis A* below the vertebra for C_6 and C_7 or above the vertebra for C_3 and C_4. Thus the axis A (fig. 47) is still **the composite axis of rotation and lateral flexion.**

An oblique radiograph of the cervical vertebral column (fig. 50) allows one to trace *the direction of the plane of the anterior facets:*

the planes a, b, c, d, e are all *oblique* anteroposteriorly;

their obliquity increases infero-superiorly. The angle between the horizontal and the line through the interspace between C_7–T_1 is only 10° while the corresponding angle for the interspaces C_2–C_3 is 40°–45°. Therefore there is an angle of 30°–35° between the lines passing through the lowest interspace f and the highest interspace a.

However, these various planes do not exactly converge at one point. The obliquity of these planes does not increase regularly in an infero-superior direction, as the three lowest planes (d, e, f) are nearly parallel, while the uppermost planes (a, b, c) are more oblique.

If one draws a *line perpendicular through the centre of each articular facet*, this line corresponds to the projection of *the axis A* of fig. 47 on to the sagittal plane. The obliquity of these axes (1–6) increases regularly but the lowest axis (6) is almost vertical indicating *almost pure rotation* at that level, while the highest axis (1) forms an angle of 40°–45° with the vertical indicating *almost equal rotation and lateral flexion* (see page 204) at that level.

Fig. 50 also shows small arrows which represent the *centres of movement*, according to Penning, and correspond to the locations *of the transverse axis of flexion and extension* of each overlying vertebra. (These centres were defined by studying lateral radiographs in extreme flexion and extension). It must be stressed that, as one approaches the base of the cervical vertebral column, these centres move upwards and forwards within the vertebral body. The position of these centres does not coincide with that determined by the intersection of the lines that pass through the centres of the inferior articular facet of the vertebra and its inferior plateau and perpendicular to their surfaces. This theoretical position is indicated by small stars.

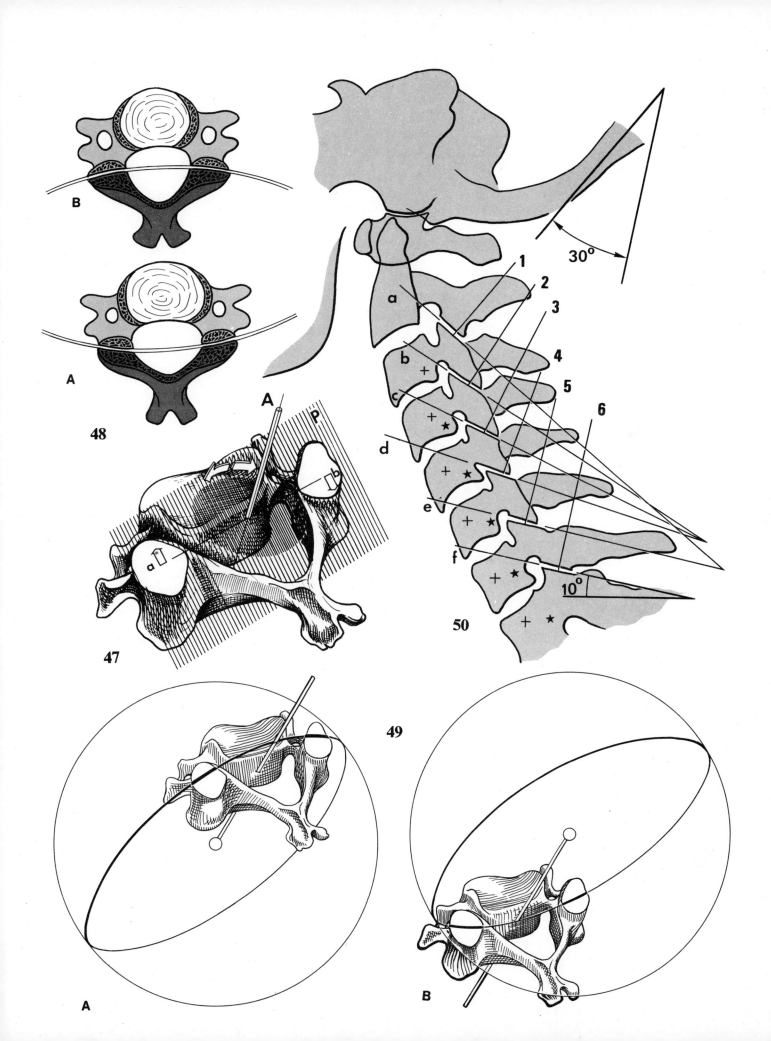

48

B

A

47

A

P

a

b

49

A

B

50

a

1

2

3

4

5

6

b

c

d

e

f

+

★

30°

10°

COMBINED LATERAL FLEXION AND ROTATION IN THE
LOWER CERVICAL VERTEBRAL COLUMN

As shown before, rotation at each segment of the column occurs about an oblique axis and is always associated with lateral flexion. If the cervical vertebral column is considered as a whole from C_2 to T_1, extension is also added to these movements (fig. 51). In fact, if one starts from T_1, which lies strictly within the axis of the column, any movement between C_7 and T_1 amounts to a mixed rotation and lateral flexion of C_7, whereas any movement between C_6 and C_7, now starting from a position of rotation and lateral flexion, is associated not only with rotation and lateral flexion but also with extension. This combination of movements becomes more significant as one passes from the lower to the upper cervical region. If this composite movement of the lower cervical vertebral column is resolved along the three planes of reference with the use of anterior and oblique radiographs (unfortunately transverse radiographs cannot be taken) it can be shown that:

the frontal plane (F) corresponds to *lateral flexion*;

the sagittal plane (S) corresponds to *extension*;

the transverse or horizontal plane (H) corresponds to *rotation*.

Therefore it can be stated that, apart from flexion and extension, the cervical vertebral column can only perform stereotyped movements of mixed lateral flexion–rotation–extension, the extension component being automatically compensated for in part by flexion in the lower part of the cervical column. On the other hand, as we shall see, the other components of this composite movement can only be compensated for at the level of the upper cervical column.

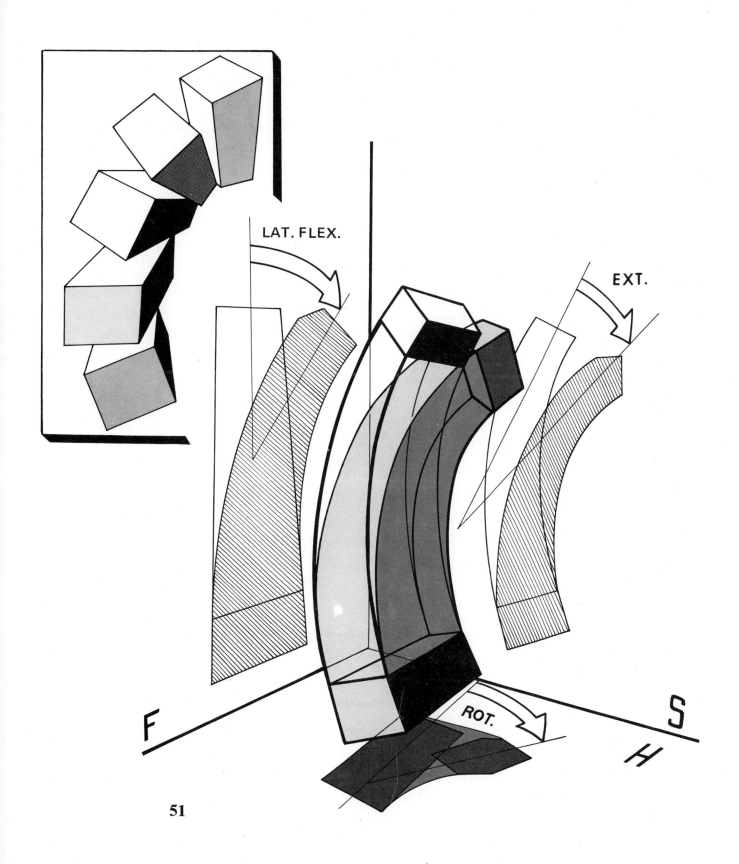

LAT. FLEX.

EXT.

ROT.

F

S

H

51

203

GEOMETRICAL ANALYSIS OF THE COMPONENTS OF
LATERAL FLEXION AND ROTATION

To grasp the mechanism of these composite movements one can make use of **a simple geometrical analysis**.

A *three-dimensional diagram* (fig. 52) allows one to imagine the movement of rotation about the axis UU′ running, like the composite axis of lateral flexion and rotation, an oblique course inferiorly and anteriorly. This axis lies in the sagittal plane formed by the vertical axis of reference ZZ′ and the horizontal axis of reference YY′. It runs towards the point of intersection of the three axes of reference, ZZ′ vertical, YY′ sagittal and XX′ transverse. If a segment OK perpendicular to the axis UU′ rotates about this axis UU′, for example to the right, it moves to OL. At the same time its projection O′M in the horizontal plane moves to O′N and similarly its projection O″K′ in the frontal plane moves to O″L′. It is possible to determine the value of the angle K′O″L′ and MO′N in terms of the angle of rotation KOL and the angle between UU′ and the vertical.

This is more easily worked out on a *simplified diagram* (fig. 53), where the axis UU′ makes an angle a with the vertical v and the segment OK represents initial position and OL the position after an angular rotation of a about the axis UU′. The angle of rotation c and the angle of lateral flexion can be calculated as follows:

$$\tan c = \frac{MN}{OM} = \frac{KL}{OM}; \qquad \tan b = \frac{KL}{OK} \quad \text{so that} \quad KL = OK \times \tan b$$

$$\cos a = \frac{OM}{OK} \quad \text{so that} \quad OM = OK \times \cos a$$

Therefore
$$\mathbf{\tan c = \frac{\tan b}{\cos a}}$$

Also
$$\sin a = \frac{KM}{OK} \quad \text{so that} \quad KM = OK \times \sin a; \qquad \tan d = \frac{KL}{KM}$$

Therefore
$$\mathbf{\tan d = \frac{\tan b}{\sin a}}$$

This analysis also allows one to study the *two extreme positions*:

if the axis UU′ is *vertical, angle a is 0°, cos a = 1*, and sin a = 0, so that tan c = tan b and angle c = angle b. Therefore when this axis UU′ is vertical *rotation about this axis is pure without any lateral flexion*;

conversely, if the axis UU′ were *horizontal* (a practical impossibility) sin a = 1 and angle d = angle b, i.e., any rotation about the axis UU′ would in fact be *pure lateral flexion*.

In the *intermediate position*, i.e., UU′ lying at an angle of 45° with the vertical, it can be shown that the angle of rotation c is equal to the angle of lateral flexion d.

Coming back to fig. 52, one notes that, when the upper vertebra rotates on the lower vertebra, through an angle KOL, it carries along with it the axis V_1 of its joint with the upper vertebra. This axis then moves to V_2 and, as it leaves the sagittal plane, it becomes *oblique with respect to the three axes of reference*, which explains the appearance of a new component of movement, i.e., extension. It would be possible to calculate the values of these angles at each segment but this would be so complicated as to require a computer. It is thus easier to understand these movements with the help of a *mechanical model*.

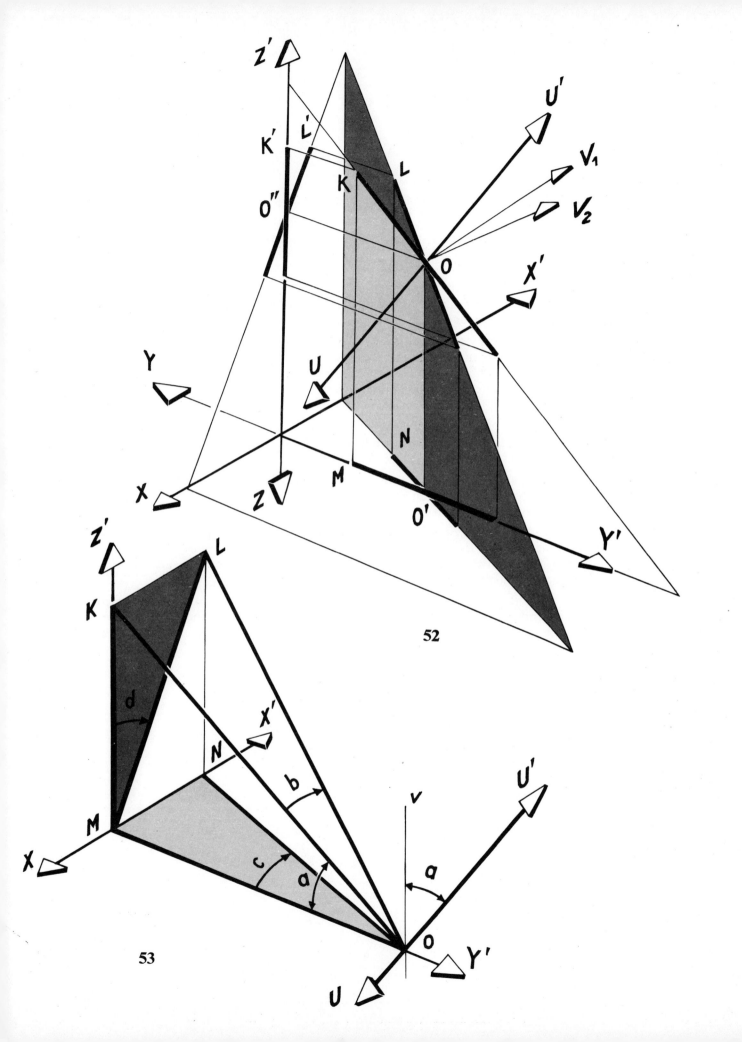

52

53

MECHANICAL MODEL OF THE CERVICAL VERTEBRAL COLUMN

From a knowledge of the structure of the vertebrae and of the functional division between the upper and lower segments of the cervical column, a mechanical model has been devised (fig. 54) which illustrates the various movements of the cervical column.

For the lower cervical column, i.e., between C_2 and T_1, only the composite movements of lateral flexion and rotation are shown occurring about *oblique axes* (see page 208) in accordance with their anatomical obliquity and their orientation relative to the vertebral bodies which, in the model, are not connected by intervertebral discs. The vertebral bodies themselves limit lateral flexion and rotation. Flexion and extension have been deliberately left out so as not to obscure the movements of lateral flexion and rotation.

The suboccipital cervical column has been built in strict accordance with its mechanical properties. It shows therefore:

a **vertical axis**, corresponding to the *odontoid*, and allowing *rotation* and some flexion and extension of the elliptical plateau representing the atlas, as a result of a certain measure of play deliberately introduced between the plateau and C_2;

a **small complex**, corresponding to the atlanto-occipital joint, with a *vertical axis* passing through the centre of the plateau of the atlas and *two axes perpendicular* to each other and to the vertical axis, corresponding to the *axes of lateral flexion and of flexion and extension* at the atlanto-occipital joint.

As a whole the suboccipital vertebral column is the equivalent of a **joint complex with three axes and three degrees of freedom** which connects C_2 to the occiput, shown in the model as a horizontal plank solidly fixed to the three main planes of reference of the head:

the sagittal plane (striped);

the frontal plane (white);

the transverse plane (striped and dark).

This model allows one to understand how the two segments of the cervical column are functionally complementary. Thus one notes that *lateral flexion and rotation to the right of the lower column is transformed into pure lateral flexion in the suboccipital segment by the loss of unwanted components.*

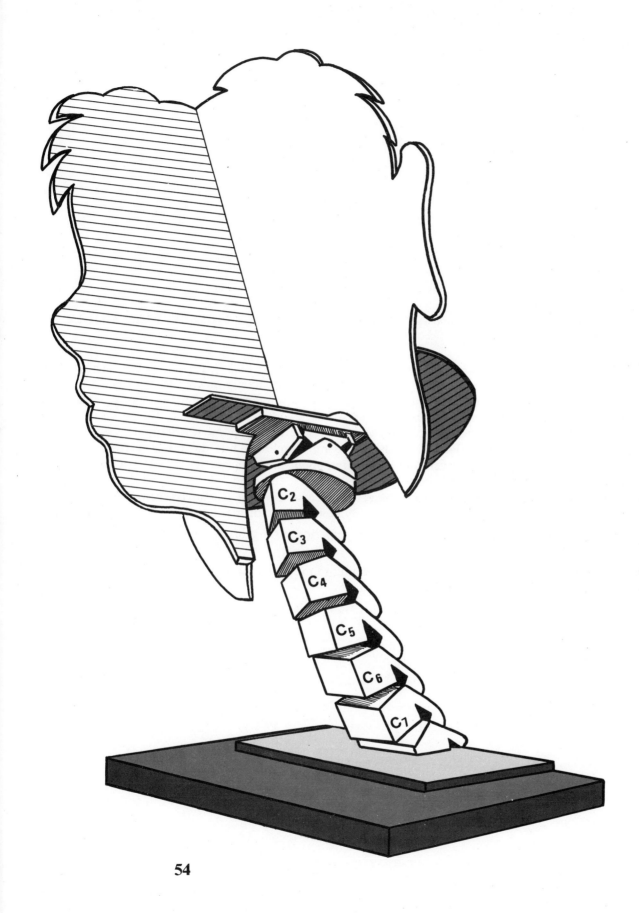

54

LATERAL FLEXION AND ROTATION ON THE MECHANICAL MODEL

If the *lower part of the cervical column is examined in detail* (fig. 53), it is clear that each posterior arch is represented functionally by a small plank lying obliquely downwards and backwards and supported on a wedge-shaped block. The role of these blocks (see fig. 50) is to reproduce the convergence of the planes of the articular surfaces and thus to simulate the cervical lordosis. The oblique axis is shown as a screw, which is attached perpendicularly to each of these surfaces and allows the locking of the overlying vertebra. Thus the upper vertebra can only move relative to the lower vertebra by rotating about this axis (see fig. 50). If one progressively rotates this six-piece model around its various axes, the model shows a *combination of lateral flexion and rotation* (fig. 56) *with a range of 50° corresponding to that of the cervical column,* as well as a slight degree of extension not easily seen in these diagrams.

One should also note the shape of the superior surface of C_2 which *functionally* represents the atlanto-axial joint:

it is *convex postero-anteriorly*, corresponding to the *superior facets of the axis* and allows flexion and extension of the atlas (not shown here);

its *vertical axis* juts out and functionally represents the *odontoid* allowing rotation to occur.

208

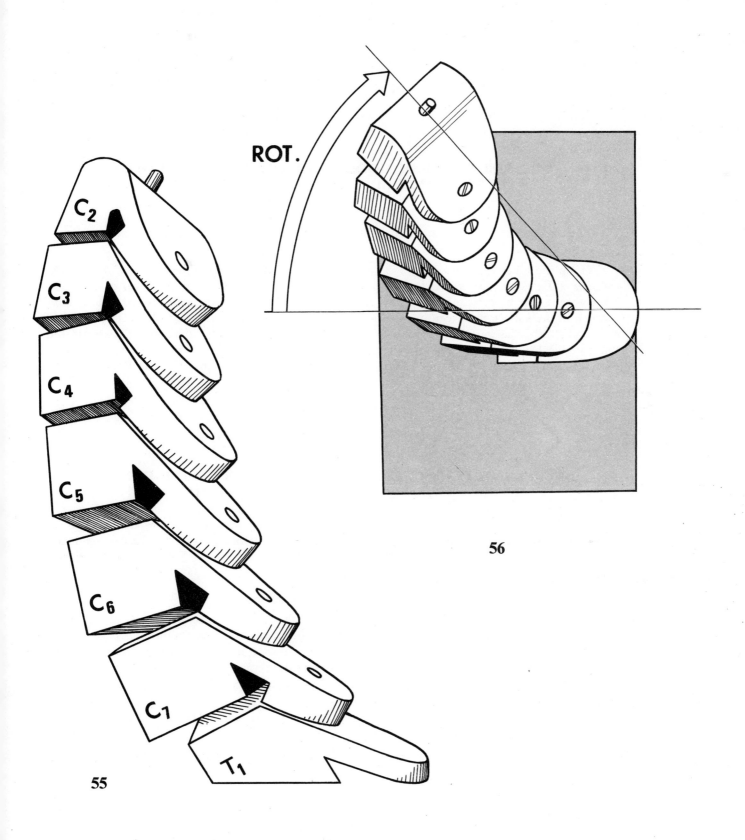

ROT.

C_2

C_3

C_4

C_5

C_6

C_7

T_1

55

56

209

COMPARISON OF THE MODEL AND THE CERVICAL COLUMN
DURING LATERAL FLEXION AND ROTATION

If the model is viewed from the front (fig. 57) it is clear that rotation of the lower cervical column to one side is associated with a lateral flexion of 25°.

If, on the other hand, a *radiograph is taken strictly in the antero-posterior plane during pure rotation of the head* (fig. 58), *a lateral flexion of 25°* is seen to occur at the level of the axis. Therefore it can be concluded that, on the one hand, *lateral flexion is always associated with rotation* in the suboccipital region (as shown by Fick and Weber at the end of the last century) and, on the other (as more recently advanced by Penning and Brugger), that *lateral flexion* in the lower cervical column is *compensated for in the suboccipital region* to produce pure rotation and, vice versa, that rotation in the lower segment is compensated for in the suboccipital segment to produce pure lateral flexion (see fig. 54).

COMPENSATIONS IN THE SUBOCCIPITAL VERTEBRAL COLUMN

A detailed view of the mechanical model (fig. 59) **in pure rotation** shows the mechanical structure of the suboccipital vertebral column as well as the compensating structures introduced to produce pure rotation.

From the top downwards the following can be seen:

the horizontal plateau (A) representing the base of the occiput;

attached to the inferior surface of the former near the front are two props (B) representing the anteroposterior axis (4) of lateral flexion at the atlanto-occipital joint. This axis (4) is connected to the intermediate piece C, which has a transverse axis (3) corresponding to the axis of flexion and extension at the atlanto-occipital joint;

this transverse axis (3) is supported by two vertical pieces (D') directly continuous with the horizontal plateau (D), which rotates on the plateau (E) with the help of a vertical axis (2) representing the axis of rotation of the atlanto-occipital joint (which is obscured by C);

the plateau E, which is functionally equivalent to the atlas, is connected to the axis (F) by a vertical piece (1) representing the odontoid and shown here as an incompletely tightened screw, which allows rotation and flexion and extension on the convex superior surface of the axis F.

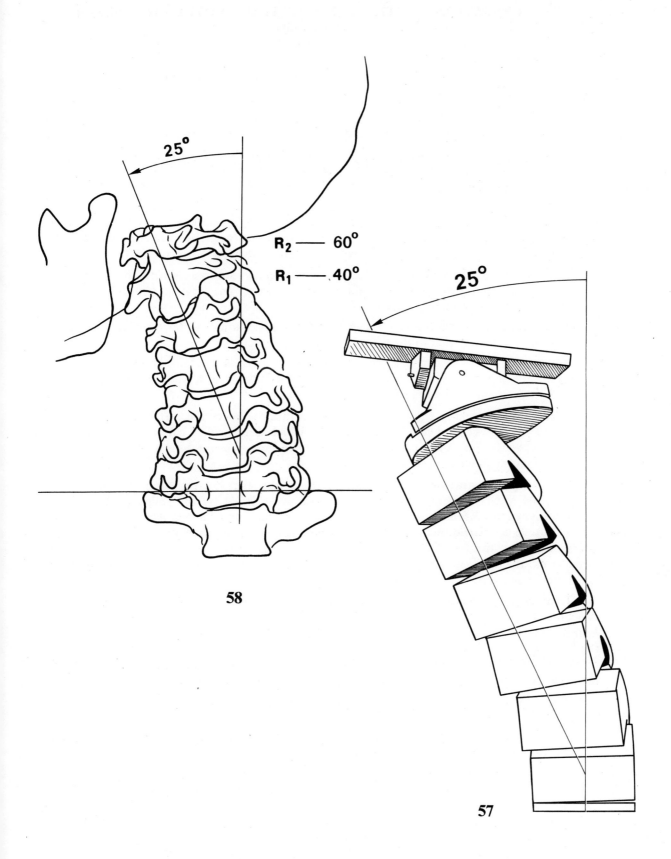

25°

R₂ — 60°

R₁ — 40°

25°

58

57

211

COMPENSATIONS IN THE SUBOCCIPITAL VERTEBRAL COLUMN
(continued)

Taken as a single anatomic entity, the suboccipital vertebral column clearly has *three functional components*:

the axis (F) with its odontoid process—axis 1;

the atlas (E) in contact with the odontoid and the superior surface of the axis;

the occiput (A) overlying a functional complex with three axes perpendicular to one another, corresponding to the axes of the atlanto-axial joint, i.e., the axis of rotation (2), the axis of flexion and extension (3) and the axis of lateral flexion (4). The last two axes interact so as to constitute a universal joint.

When lateral flexion and rotation occur simultaneously in the lower cervical column, pure rotation of the occiput is achieved by the following **three movements** which must occur at the suboccipital joint complex with its three axes and its three degrees of freedom:

rotation to the right, about axes 1 and 2, is functionally continuous with that of the lower cervical column and takes place largely at the atlanto-axial joint (angle a) and to a lesser extent at the atlanto-occipital joint (angle b);

extension occurring about the axis 3 (angle c) and compensating for flexion which would occur as a result of pure rotation to the right about axis 1;

finally a small degree of *lateral flexion in the opposite direction* (angle d) about the axis 4, since most of the lateral flexion of the lower cervical column has already been neutralised by extension occurring about axis 3.

Anatomically speaking, these movements occur in the suboccipital vertebral column with the help of the *small suboccipital muscles* (see page 232) which can be called collectively the **fine tuner** since their essential function is to *adjust finely the compensatory movements* so that only the wanted component of any movement is retained.

During pure rotation of the head to the right (fig. 59), the complementary rotation of the suboccipital vertebral column to the right is achieved by the following muscles—the *right obliquus capitis inferior* and *rectus capitis posterior major* and the *left obliquus capitis superior*. These muscles all extend the head and bring about the extension mentioned above. The contralateral flexion to the left is achieved by the *left obliquus capitis superior*, the *left rectus capitis lateralis* and the *left rectus capitis posterior minor*. The flexion achieved by the latter two muscles is counterbalanced by the extension brought about by the former muscles.

During pure lateral flexion of the head to the right (fig. 54) *counter-rotation to the left* is achieved by the following muscles—the *left obliquus superior and the two posterior recti* and *lateral flexion to the right by the two posterior recti and the inferior oblique on the right side*. Finally the extension caused by these muscles as well as the extension in the lower cervical column and the extension that would follow counter-rotation to the left are compensated for by the flexor muscles: the *right rectus capitis anterior* and the *rectus capitis lateralis*.

Thus this mechanical model allows one to understand the anatomical and functional connection between:

on the one hand, the **lower cervical vertebral column**, which shows a composite movement of rotation, lateral flexion and extension. It is equipped with muscles ideally disposed for this type of movement, i.e., long muscles running an oblique course posteriorly, laterally and inferiorly, like the splenius cervicis, the longissimus capitis, the intertransverse muscles, the iliocostalis, the levator scapulae and to a lesser degree the scalene muscles;

on the other, the **suboccipital vertebral column** which consists of a *joint complex with three axes and three degrees of freedom* and controlled by the *fine tuning of the suboccipital muscles* which, by their synergistic-antagonistic action, can eliminate at the level of the suboccipital joints unwanted components of movement deriving from the lower cervical column and thus produce any pure movement.

212

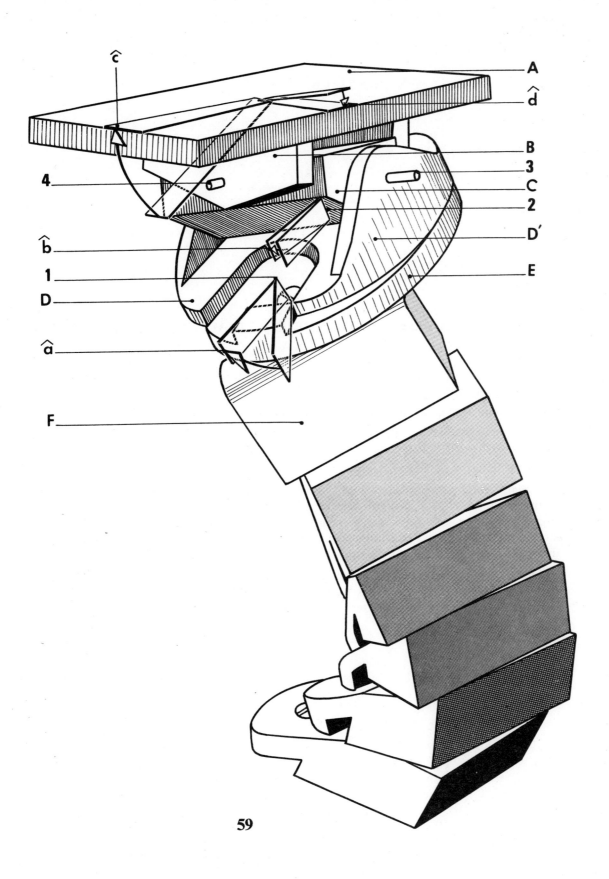

Ĉ

A

d̂

B

3

4

C

2

D′

b̂

1

E

D

â

F

59

213

RANGE OF MOVEMENTS OF THE CERVICAL VERTEBRAL COLUMN

By studying *oblique radiographs* taken in the extreme positions of **flexion and extension** (fig. 60) it has been established that:

the total range of flexion and extension *in the lower cervical column* is 100–110° (LCC);

the total range of flexion and extension *for the whole cervical column* (WC) is 130° with reference to the plane of the bite;

by subtraction, the range of flexion and extension in the *suboccipital column* (SO) is 20–30°.

Similarly *anteroposterior views* with the head in extreme positions of lateral flexion (fig. 61) show that the total range of **lateral flexion** is about 45°. By drawing, on the one hand, the line joining the two transverse processes of the atlas and, on the other, the line joining the base of the mastoid processes one can deduce that the range of lateral flexion is about 8° in the suboccipital column, i.e., *occurring solely at the atlanto-occipital joint*.

The range of **rotation** is more difficult to evaluate, especially as regards its various segmental components (fig. 62). The total range of rotation of the head varies from 80–90° on either side. It amounts to 12° at the *atlanto-occipital joint* and at the *atlanto-axial joint*.

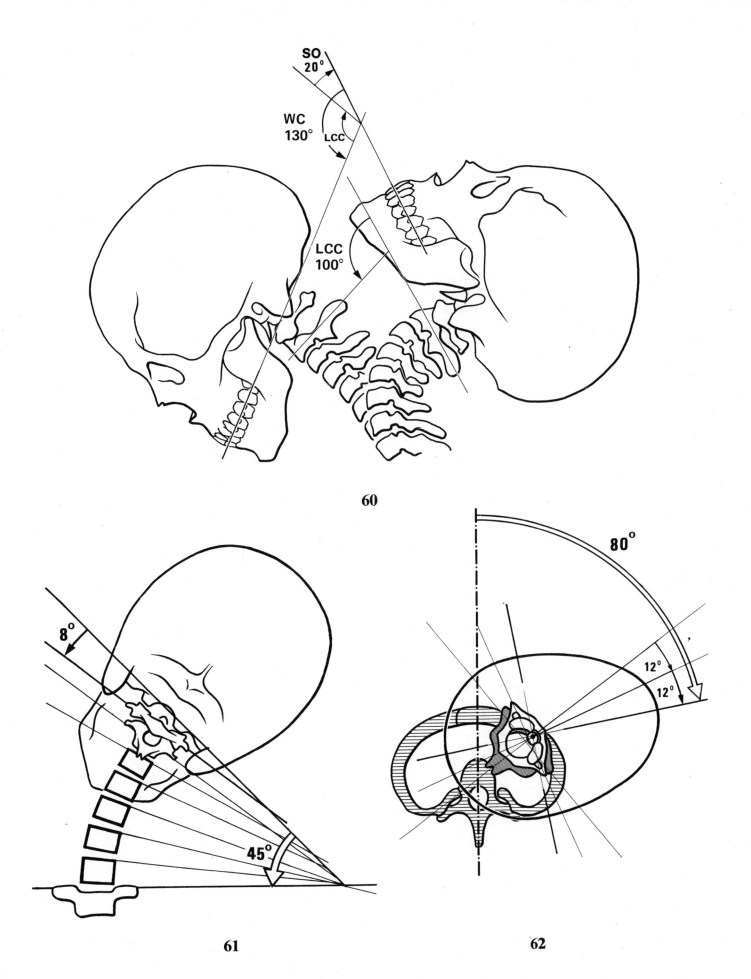

60

61

62

THE BALANCING OF THE HEAD ON THE CERVICAL VERTEBRAL COLUMN

The head is in equilibrium (fig. 63) when the *eyes look horizontally*. In this position the *plane of the bite* (B), shown here by a piece of cardboard held tightly between the teeth, is also horizontal as is the *auriculo-nasal plane* (AN), which passes through the nasal spine and the superior border of the external auditory meatus.

The head taken as a whole constitutes a *lever system*:

the *fulcrum* O lies at the level of the occipital condyles;

the *force* G is produced by the weight of the head applied through its centre of gravity lying near the sella turcica;

the *force* F is produced by the posterior neck muscles which constantly counterbalance the weight of the head, which tends to tilt it forwards.

This anterior location of the centre of gravity of the head explains the strength of the posterior neck muscles relative to the flexor muscles of the neck. In fact the *extensor muscles counteract gravity* whereas the flexors are helped by gravity. This also explains the constant tone in these posterior neck muscles preventing the head from tilting forwards. When one sleeps while sitting the tone of these muscles is reduced and the head falls on the chest.

The cervical vertebral column is not straight but is concave posteriorly, i.e., a **cervical lordosis** which can be characterised by:

the *chord subtending the arc* (C) running in a straight line from the basi-occiput to the postero-inferior corners of C_7;

the *perpendicular* (P) joining the mid-point of the chord C to the apex of the curve and touching the postero-inferior border of C_4.

This latter parameter increases with accentuation of the cervical lordosis and equals zero when the cervical column is straight. It can even become negative when during flexion the cervical column becomes concave anteriorly. This chord is always smaller than the full length of the cervical column and only equals it when the cervical column is straight. Thus a *cervical index* could be established along the lines of the Delmas Index (page 20).

216

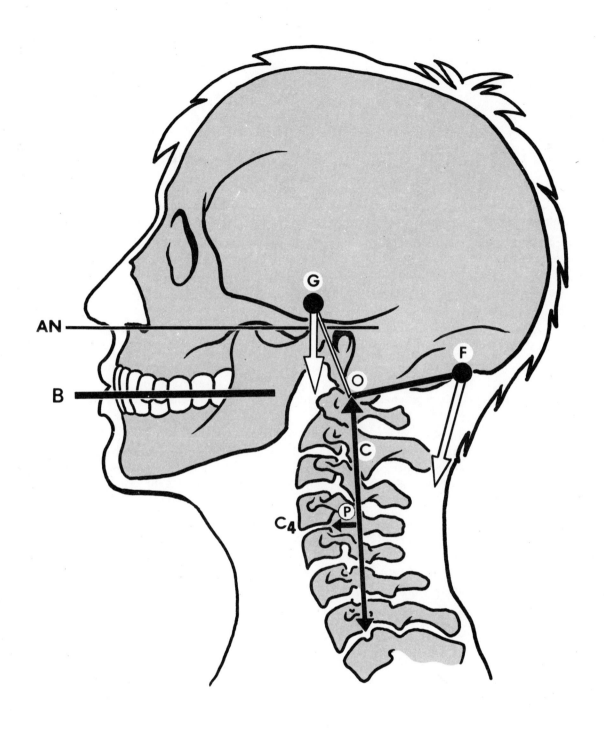

63

217

STRUCTURE AND ACTION OF THE STERNO-CLEIDO-MASTOID

This muscle should be called the sterno-cleido-occipito-mastoid (S.C.O.M.) as it is made up of **four distinct bands** (fig. 75):

a deep band, the *cleido-mastoid* (CM) running from the medial third of the clavicle to the mastoid process;

three superficial bands which can be teased out into a N shape, though they are normally closely interwoven except in their infero-medial part near the medial end of the clavicle. These three superficial bands are:

the *cleido-occipital* which overlies the bulk of the cleido-mastoid and is inserted into the lateral third of the superior nuchal line of the occipital;

the *sterno-occipital* and the *sterno-mastoid*, both of which arise by a common tendon from the superior margin of the sternum. The sterno-occipital is inserted along with the cleido-occipital into the superior nuchal line, while the sterno-mastoid is inserted into the superior and anterior borders of the mastoid.

Taken as a whole the S.C.O.M. forms a large muscular band which runs obliquely downwards and forwards on the antero-lateral aspect of the neck. Its most conspicuous portion is the common tendon of the sterno-occipital and sterno-mastoid, which two muscles constitute a fusiform muscle mass easily visible under the skin. These two tendons right and left bound the suprasternal notch.

Unilateral contraction of this muscle (fig. 65) gives rise to a triple movement combining rotation of the head contralaterally, lateral flexion ipsilaterally and extension. This position of the head is typical of congenital torticollis, very often due to one short S.C.O.M.

The effects of *bilateral contraction* of the two S.C.O.M. will be discussed later. These effects vary according to the state of contraction of the other neck muscles:

if the cervical vertebral column is *flexible*, this bilateral contraction *accentuates the cervical lordosis with extension of the head* and flexion of the cervical column relative to the thoracic column (see fig. 92);

if, on the contrary, the cervical column is kept *straight and rigid* by the contraction of the prevertebral muscles, then bilateral contraction produces *flexion of the cervical column relative to the thoracic column* and *forward flexion of the head* (see fig. 97).

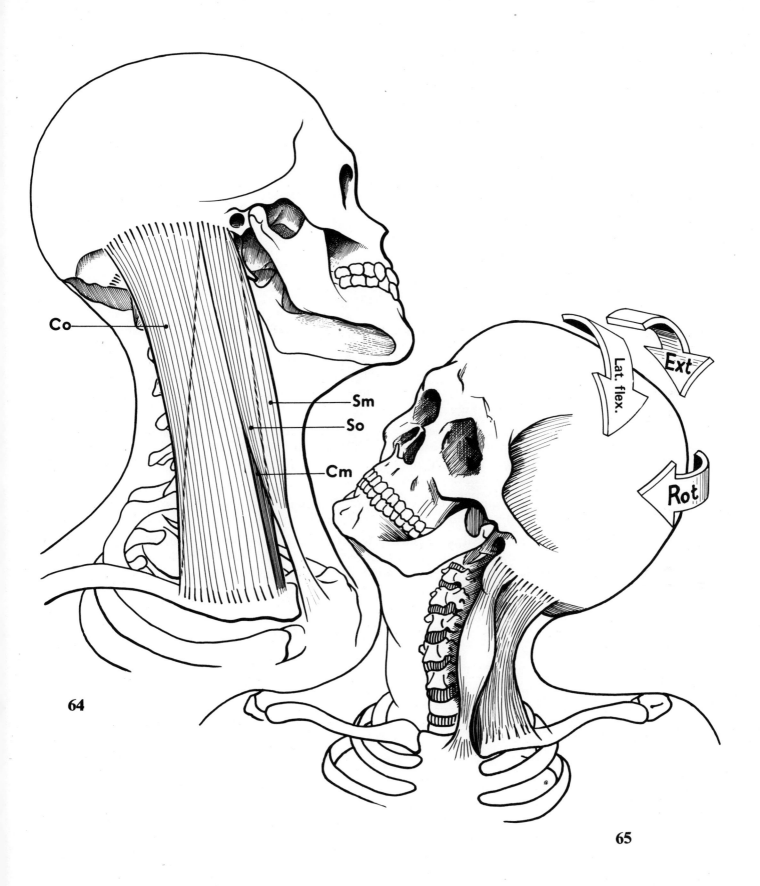

Co

Sm
So

Cm

64

Lat. flex.

Ext

Rot

65

THE PREVERTEBRAL MUSCLES: THE LONGUS CERVICIS

The longus cervicis (l.c.) is the *deepest of the prevertebral muscles* (fig. 66) and runs on the anterior surface of the cervical column from the superior arch of the atlas to the third thoracic vertebra. It consists of three sets of fibres anatomically:

an *oblique descending set* attached to the anterior tubercle of the atlas and to the anterior tubercle of the transverse process of C_3–C_6 by three or four tendinous slips;

an *oblique ascending set* attached to the bodies of T_2 and T_3 and to the anterior tubercle of the transverse process of C_4–C_7 by three or four tendinous slips;

a *longitudinal set* lying deep to the former two sets and just lateral to the midline. It is attached to the bodies of the first three thoracic vertebrae and the last six cervical vertebrae.

Thus the longus cervicis, on either side of the midline, covers the whole anterior surface of the cervical column. When *both muscles contract symmetrically* they flatten the cervical curvature and flex the neck. They are also important in stabilising the cervical column at rest.

Contraction of one longus cervicis produces forward and lateral flexion of the cervical column ipsilaterally.

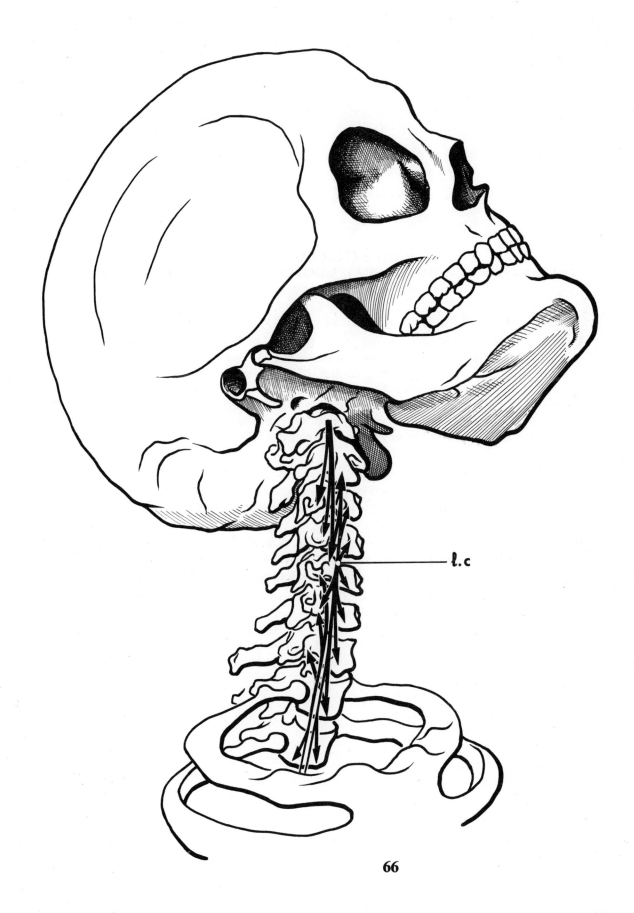

ℓ.c

66

THE PREVERTEBRAL MUSCLES:
THE ANTERIOR AND LATERAL RECTUS MUSCLES OF THE NECK

These muscles belong to the upper reaches of the cervical vertebral column (fig. 67).

The **rectus capitis anterior** consists of two bands. The **deep band** (also called the *rectus capitis anterior major*—R.A.Ma.) is the most median muscle and touches its homologue on the other side. It is attached to the inferior surface of the basi-occiput anterior to the foramen magnum and to the anterior tubercles of the transverse processes of C_3–C_6, and overlies the longus cervicis. It acts on the suboccipital vertebral column and on the upper part of the lower cervical column. *Bilateral contraction* produces *flexion of the head* on the cervical column and a flattening of the lordosis of the upper portion of the cervical column. *Unilateral contraction* causes *forward and lateral flexion* of the head ipsilaterally.

The **superficial band** (also called the *rectus capitis anterior minor*—R.A.Mi.) lies posterior and lateral to the former and stretches from the basi-occiput to the anterior aspect of the lateral mass of the atlas up to the anterior tubercle of its transverse process. It runs obliquely inferiorly and laterally.

Bilateral contraction of these muscles produces *flexion of the head* on the cervical column at the level of the atlanto-occipital joint. *Unilateral contraction* produces a *triple movement combining forward flexion, rotation* and *lateral flexion ipsilaterally*, and occurring at the atlanto-occipital joint.

The **rectus capitis lateralis** (r.l.) is the highest of the intertransverse muscles and is attached to the jugular process of the occiput and to the anterior tubercle of the transverse process of the atlas. It lies lateral to the anterior rectus and overlies the anterior surface of the atlanto-occipital joint. Its *bilateral contraction* produces *flexion* of the head on the cervical column; its *unilateral contraction* produces a *slight lateral flexion* of the head *ipsilaterally*. Both these movements occur at the atlanto-occipital joint.

222

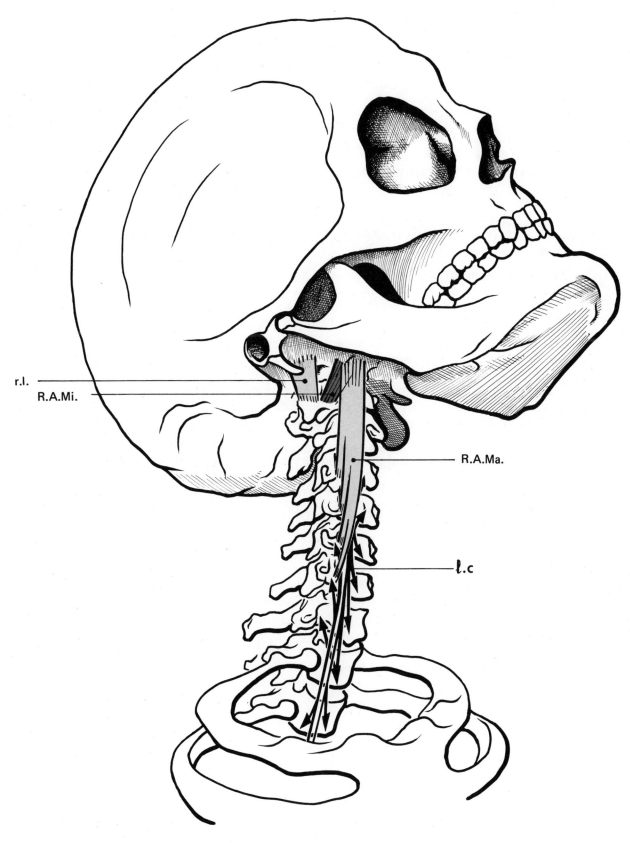

r.l.

R.A.Mi.

R.A.Ma.

ℓ.c

67

THE PREVERTEBRAL MUSCLES: THE SCALENE MUSCLES

The three scalene muscles lie on the antero-lateral aspect of the cervical vertebral column like *muscular tighteners* (fig. 68) and connect the transverse processes of the vertebrae to the first two ribs.

The **scalenus anterior** (s.a.) is triangular with its apex lying inferiorly and takes origin from the anterior tubercles of the transverse processes of C_3–C_6. Its fibres converge down to be inserted by a tendon into the scalene tubercle on the superior aspect of the first rib. Its fibres as a whole run an oblique course inferiorly, anteriorly and laterally.

The **scalenus medius** (s.m.) lies in contact with the deep surface of the former and arises by tendinous slips from the posterior tubercles of the transverse processes of C_2–C_7, the lateral edge of the gutter-like depression in the transverse processes of C_2–C_6 and the transverse process of C_7. The muscle is flattened anteroposteriorly and triangular with its apex located inferiorly. Its fibres run obliquely, inferiorly, laterally and slightly anteriorly to be inserted into the superior surface of the first rib just posterior to the groove for the subclavian artery.

The **scalenus posterior** (s.p.) lies posterior to the other two. It arises by three tendinous slips from the posterior tubercles of the transverse processes of C_4–C_6. It is flattened transversely and lies lateral and posterior to the scalenus medius, with which it is more or less continuous. It is inserted by a flat tendon into the superior border and the lateral aspect of the second rib.

Between the anterior and middle scalenes run the *roots of the brachial plexus and the subclavian artery*.

When *these muscles contract symmetrically the cervical column is flexed on the thoracic column* and the *cervical lordosis is accentuated* if the neck is not held rigid by contraction of the longus cervicis. On the other hand, if the cervical column is *held rigid* by the longus cervicis, symmetrical contraction of the scalenes can *only flex* the cervical column on the thoracic column (see fig. 93).

If the *scalenes contract only on one side* the cervical column is *laterally flexed* and *rotated* towards the side of their contraction.

They are also accessory inspiratory muscles as they can elevate the first two ribs when their cervical vertebral attachments are kept steady.

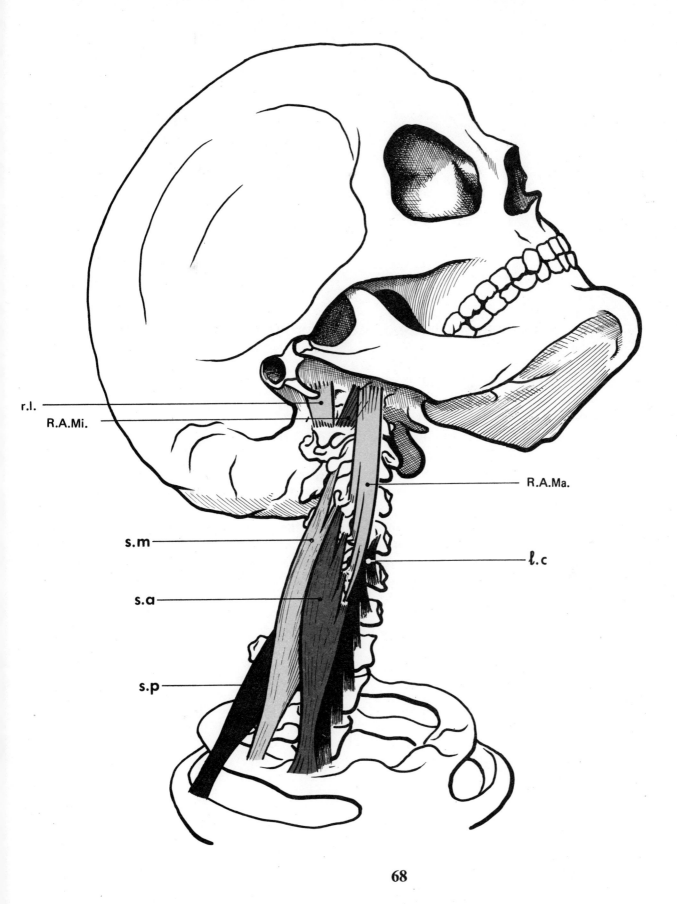

r.l.

R.A.Mi.

R.A.Ma.

s.m

ℓ.c

s.a

s.p

68

THE PREVERTEBRAL MUSCLES VIEWED AS A WHOLE

Using Testut's diagram (fig. 69) it is possible to localise at once **all the prevertebral muscles**:

the *longus cervicis* (l.c.) with its longitudinal fibres (1) and its ascending (a.o.) and descending (d.o.) oblique fibres;

the *rectus capitis anterior* with its superficial (R.A.Mi.) and deep (R.A.Ma.) fibres;

the *rectus capitis lateralis* (r.l.);

the *intertransverse muscles* lying in two planes: anterior (i.t.a.) and posterior (i.t.p.). Their only action is to flex the cervical column ipsilaterally (fig. 70), with the help of the ipsilateral scalene muscles;

the *scalenus anterior* (s.a.), drawn in toto only on the right side and with its tendon left in place on the left to reveal the *scalenus medius* (s.m.);

the *scalenus posterior* (s.p.) which projects beyond the scalenus medius only in its lower part near its insertion into the second rib.

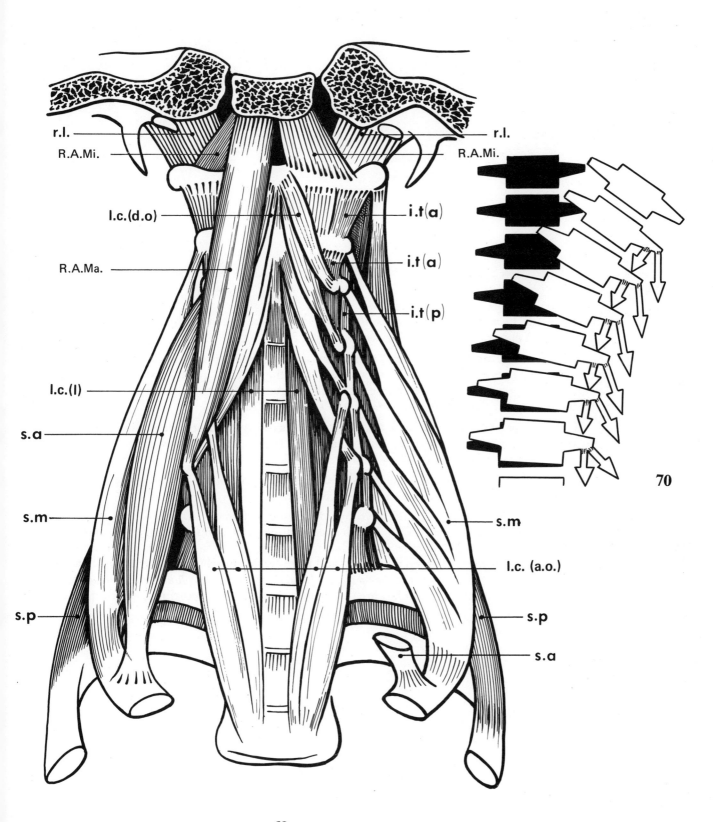

r.l.

R.A.Mi.

l.c.(d.o)

R.A.Ma.

l.c.(l)

s.a

s.m

s.p

r.l.

R.A.Mi.

i.t(a)

i.t(a)

i.t(p)

s.m

l.c. (a.o.)

s.p

s.a

69

70

FLEXION OF THE HEAD AND NECK

Flexion of the head on the cervical column and flexion of the neck on the thoracic column depend on the anterior muscles of the neck.

In the suboccipital region (fig. 71) the rectus anterior (r.a.) produces flexion at the atlanto-occipital joint. The longus cervicis ($l.c_1$ and $l.c_2$) and the anterior rectus produce *flexion* at the lower vertebral joints. It must be stressed that the longus cervicis plays the most important role in *straightening the cervical column and holding it rigid* (fig. 72).

The *anterior muscles of the neck* (fig. 73) are **located at a distance from the cervical column** and thus act via the long arm of a lever. Hence they are powerful flexors of the head and of the cervical column. They are:

the **supra-hyoid muscles**, i.e., the *mylo-hyoid* and the *anterior belly of the digastric* (not shown here) which connect the mandible and the hyoid bone;

the **infra-hyoid muscles**, i.e., the thyrohyoid, the sterno-hyoid (s.h.), the sterno-thyroid (not shown here), the omo-hyoid (o.h.). When these muscles act simultaneously the mandible is lowered but *if the mandible is fixed by contraction of the muscles of mastication*, i.e., the masseter (M) and the temporalis (T), then the supra- and infra-hyoid muscles produce *flexion of the head on the cervical column and flexion of the cervical column on the thoracic column* while *simultaneously flattening the cervical curvature*. They are thus very important in supporting the cervical column at rest.

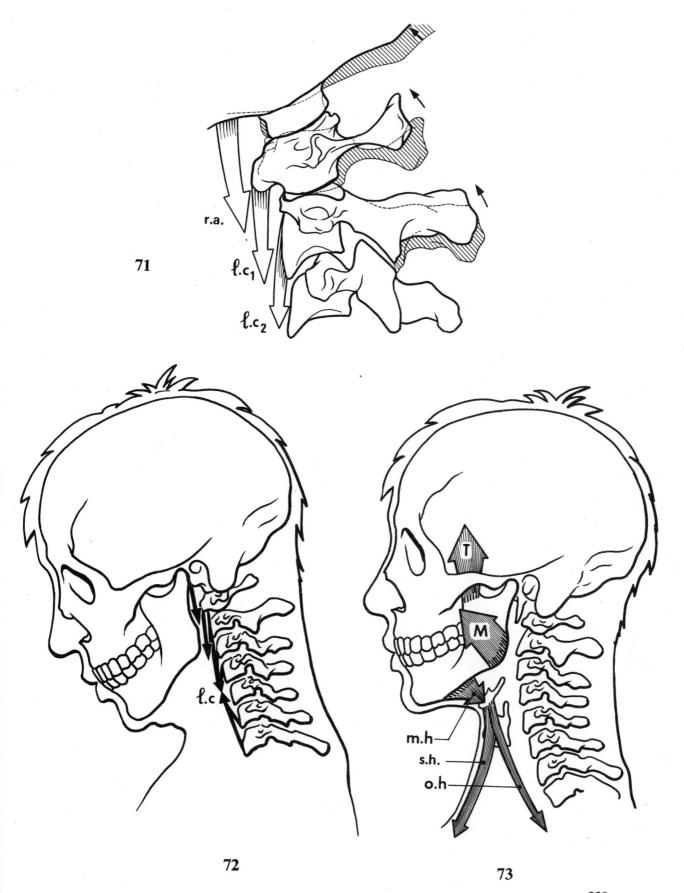

71

r.a.

ℓ.c₁

ℓ.c₂

72

ℓ.c

73

T

M

m.h

s.h.

o.h

229

THE POSTERIOR MUSCLES OF THE NECK

Before studying the action of these muscles it is essential to have a full grasp of their distribution. In fig. 74 (seen in perspective) the neck is seen from the right side and from the back and the superficial muscles have been removed to reveal the various planes.

The back of the neck is made up of *four muscular planes superimposed on one another*, as follows:

the **deep plane**, directly adherent to the vertebral bones and joints, containing—

the small intrinsic muscles of the suboccipital vertebral column running between the occiput, the atlas and the axis, i.e., the *rectus capitis posterior major* (1) and *minor* (2), the *obliquus capitis superior* (3) and *inferior* (4);

the *cervical transverso-spinalis* (5);

the *interspinous muscles* (6);

the **semispinalis plane** (partly sectioned) contains—

the *semispinalis capitis* (7) and the *semispinalis cervicis* (8);

laterally, the *transversus thoracis*, the *longissimus thoracis and the superior portion of the iliocostalis* (11);

the **plane of the splenius and the levator scapulae** (also partly sectioned) can be subdivided into two layers—

the *splenius capitis* (9);

the *splenius cervicis* (10), showing only one of its three tendons of insertion into the posterior tubercle of the transverse process of C_3 (the other two tendons of insertion into the posterior tubercles of the transverse processes of C_1 and C_2 have been removed);
the *levator scapulae* (12);
These muscles are closely moulded on to those of the deep plane, around which they wrap themselves as around a pulley (according to Florent). Thus, when they contract, they also *produce rotation* of the head;

the **superficial plane** is comprised of—

the *trapezius* (fig. 15), which has been almost completely removed here;

the *sterno-cleido-mastoid* which belongs to the posterior neck only in its postero-superior part. It is shown here partially sectioned to reveal its *superficial* (14) and its *deep cleido-mastoid* (14′) components.

In the depth of the figure, through the gap between the muscles one can see the attachments of the *scalenus medius and posterior* (13).

On the whole, except for the deep muscles, the majority of these muscles are oblique inferiorly, medially and posteriorly and so produce simultaneously *extension, rotation* and *lateral flexion towards the side of their contraction*, i.e., exactly the *three components of the composite movement of the cervical column about oblique axes* (see page 200). The superficial muscles, on the other hand, run in a counter direction to the intermediate muscles, i.e., inferiorly, anteriorly and laterally. Thus they produce extension and lateral flexion ipsilaterally, like the deeper muscles, but *rotation contralaterally*. They are therefore at once agonists and antagonists of the deeper muscles, to which they are functionally complementary.

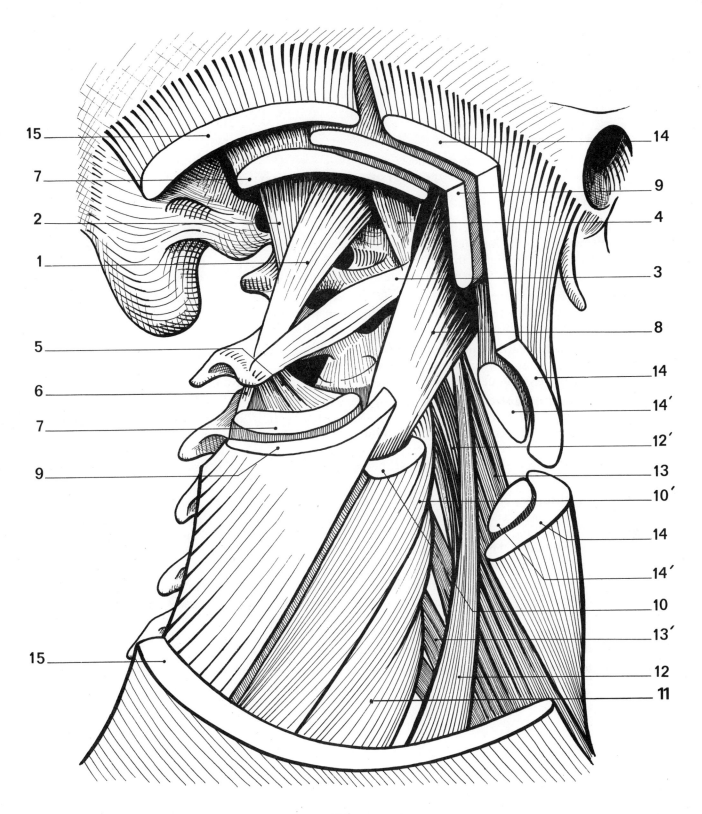

15

7

2

1

5

6

7

9

15

14

9

4

3

8

14

14´

12´

13

10´

14

14´

10

13´

12

11

74

THE SUBOCCIPITAL MUSCLES

The physiology of these muscles is usually neglected because they are not considered as complementary to the muscles of the lower cervical column. In fact, these muscles of **fine tuning** are vital in determining the position of the head by reinforcing wanted or eliminating unwanted components of the composite triple movement of the lower cervical column.

Before studying their function, it is wise to review their anatomy, particularly *their orientation in space* and this can be done by viewing them from the back (fig. 75), from the side (fig. 76) and from the right side and from below (fig. 77). These figures show:

the **rectus capitis posterior major** (1), which is triangular in shape with its base located superiorly. It is attached to the spinous process of the axis and the inferior nuchal line of the occiput. Its oblique fibres run superiorly, and slightly laterally and posteriorly;

the **rectus capitis posterior minor** (2), which is triangular, flattened and smaller than the major to which it lies deep. It lies closer to the midline and is attached to the tubercle of the posterior arch of the atlas and to the medial third of the inferior nuchal line of the occiput. Its oblique fibres run superiorly, slightly laterally and *more directly posteriorly than the rectus major*. This is due to the fact that the posterior arch of the atlas lies deeper than the spinous process of the axis;

the **obliquus capitis inferior** (3), which is an elongated, thick and fusiform muscle lying inferior and lateral to the rectus capitis major. It is attached to the lower border of the spine of the axis and to the posterior margin of the transverse process of the atlas. Its oblique fibres run superiorly, laterally and *anteriorly* and thus cross in space the above-mentioned muscles, particularly the rectus capitis posterior minor;

the **obliquus capitis superior** (4), which is a short, flattened triangular muscle lying posterior to the atlanto-occipital joint. It is attached to the transverse process of the atlas and to the lateral third of the inferior nuchal line of the occiput. Its oblique fibres run superiorly and *posteriorly*, and almost in a saggital plane as they do not run laterally at all. It lies parallel to the rectus posterior minor and perpendicular to the inferior oblique;

the **interspinous muscles** (5) lie on either side of the midline between the spines of C_3–C_7. Thus they are homologous to the two posterior rectus muscles.

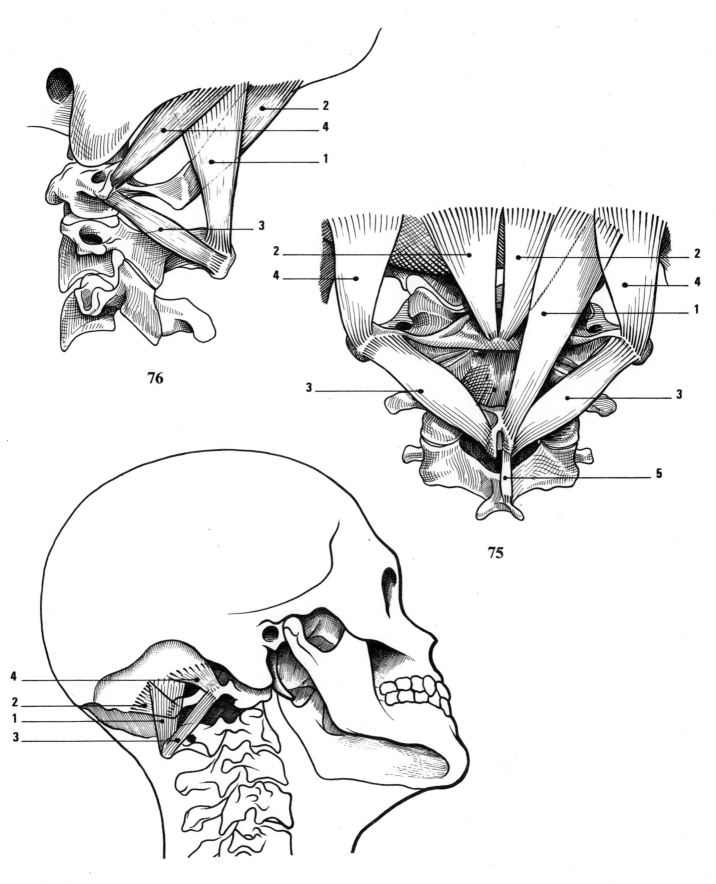

76

75

77

ACTIONS OF THE SUBOCCIPITAL MUSCLES: LATERAL FLEXION AND EXTENSION

The **obliquus capitis inferior**, as a result of its location, *is important in maintaining the integrity of the atlanto-axial joint at rest and during movements*. When seen from the side (fig. 78), this muscle pulls back the transverse processes of the atlas and so, when the two obliques contract symmetrically, they *pull back and extend the atlas on the axis*. The extension can be measured on oblique radiographs as the angle of displacement of the lateral masses of the atlas (a). When the joint is viewed from above (fig. 79), each muscle is seen as the chord that subtends an arc of a circle. When they *contract symmetrically* they pull the axis forward and as a result the atlas moves backwards over a distance r. This *relieves the tension in the transverse ligament*, which passively holds the odontoid and prevents its posterior dislocation. Thus these two muscles acting simultaneously are essential in maintaining the integrity of the atlanto-odontoid joint during activity.

Unilateral contraction of the four suboccipital muscles (fig. 80) produces *lateral flexion* of the head (arrow i) ipsilaterally at the atlanto-occipital joint. This angle of lateral flexion i is also equal to the angle i' lying between the horizontal line joining the transverse processes of the atlas and the oblique line joining the tips of the mastoid processes. The most efficient of these muscles is the *superior oblique* whose contraction increases the length of its contralateral homologue by e. Its origin is the transverse process of the atlas which is stabilised by the inferior oblique. The rectus posterior major (1) is less efficient than the superior oblique and the efficiency of the rectus minor is minimal as it lies too close to the midline.

Bilateral simultaneous contraction of the suboccipital muscles (fig. 81) produces *extension* of the head on the upper cervical column at the atlanto-occipital joint, the muscles involved being the rectus posterior minor (2) and the superior oblique (4). At the atlanto-axial joint the muscles involved are the rectus posterior major (1) and the inferior oblique (3) (fig. 78).

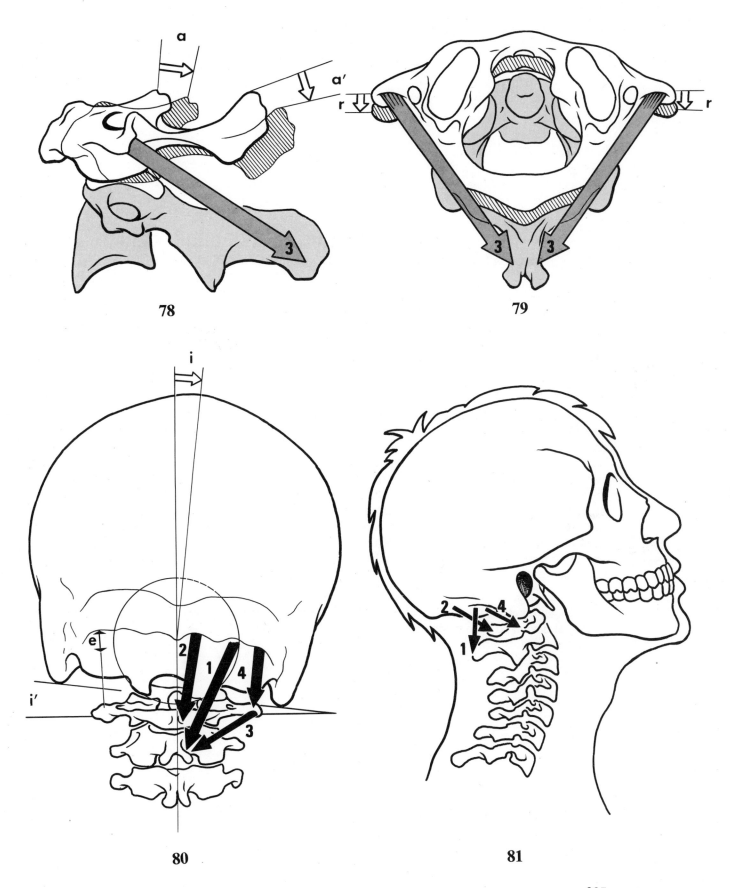

78

79

80

81

ROTATORY ACTION OF THE SUBOCCIPITAL MUSCLES

In addition to extension and lateral flexion, these muscles also *produce rotation of the head*.

Let us first consider the **atlanto-occipital joint** (fig. 82, seen from below). It is clear that the superior oblique (4) produces a 10° rotation of the head *contralaterally*, i.e., in the diagram the left superior oblique rotates the head to the right. This passively stretches the inferior oblique (4) and the rectus posterior minor (2) on the right side and these muscles restore the head to the neutral position.

Let us now consider the **atlanto-axial** joint (fig. 83, seen from below with the axis transparent and the atlas striped grey). It is clear that contraction of the rectus posterior major (1) and the inferior oblique (3) produces rotation of the head *ipsilaterally*, i.e., in the diagram the right rectus major (1) produces rotation of the head to the right both at the atlanto-occipital and the atlanto-axial joints. This passively stretches the left rectus major (a) and this muscle will restore the head to the neutral position. Contraction of the right inferior oblique (3) causes rotation of the head to the right only at the atlanto-axial joint. In an oblique view taken in perspective (fig. 84), the inferior oblique is seen running diagonally between the spine of the axis and the right transverse process of the atlas and its contraction rotates the atlas to the right while stretching the left inferior oblique by a distance b. The latter muscle will restore the head to the neutral position.

After understanding all the actions of the suboccipital muscles one should go back to page 212 so as to get a better grasp of their function in eliminating the unwanted components of rotation or lateral flexion so as to ensure pure movements of the head.

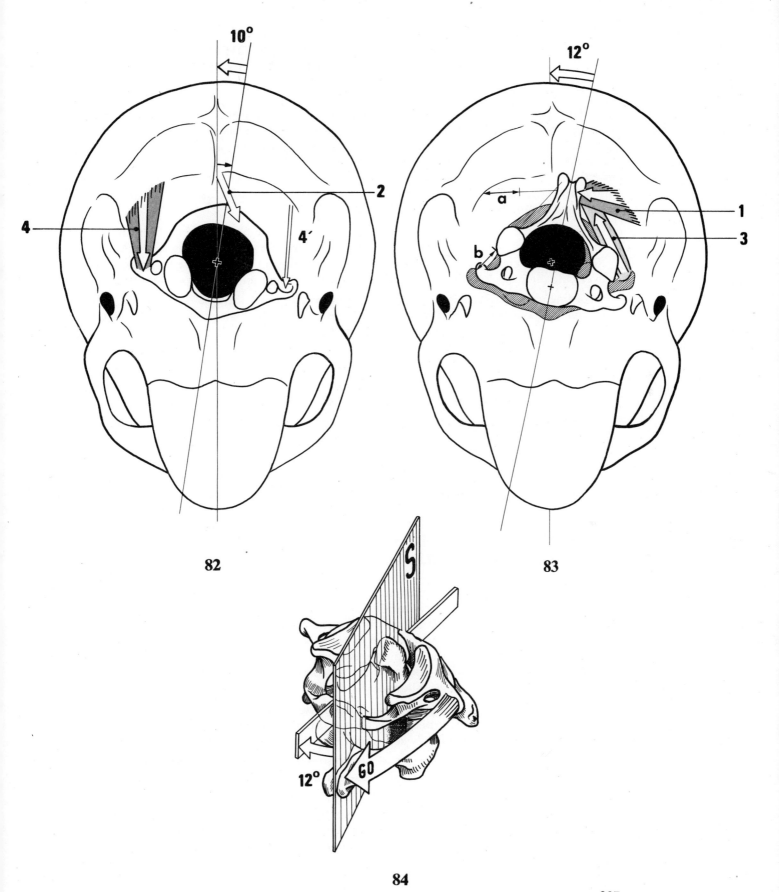

82

83

84

THE POSTERIOR MUSCLES OF THE NECK:
THE DEEP AND SUPERFICIAL PLANES

The **deep plane** consists of *the suboccipital muscles* in the upper cervical region and of *the transversospinalis muscles* in the lower cervical region. These muscles are closely adherent to the vertebrae and fill the groove formed by the spines, the laminae and the transverse processes. They are made up of *muscular slips that overhang one another like tiles on a roof.* Therefore on either side of the interspinous line there is a transversospinalis muscle filling the vertebral groove from the axis to the sacrum. The arrangement of the muscular slips has been variously interpreted by different authors (fig. 85):

according to the classic view of TROLARD (T), the muscle fibres running from the spines and the laminae of C_2–C_5 converge on to the transverse process of C_6. In the diagram (fig. 85; T) the first complete set of muscle fibres is seen inserting into the transverse process of C_6 and overlying the partial tendinous slips converging on to the transverse processes of C_3–C_5;

according to WINCKLER (W), the muscle fibres run in the inverse direction (W). They run as four muscular slips from the lamina and the spine of the highest vertebra to the transverse processes of the underlying four vertebrae. In the diagram the uppermost fibres system is shown which runs from the axis and overlies more or less the lower fibre systems.

These two theories in fact describe the same anatomical fact depending on whether the superior or the inferior end of the muscle is taken as the starting point. However, as the fibres always run an *oblique course inferiorly, laterally and slightly anteriorly*, their contraction produces:

when the muscles contract bilaterally and symmetrically, extension of the cervical column and accentuation of the cervical lordosis; therefore they are equivalent to an *erector spinae cervicis*;

when only one muscle contracts, lateral flexion ipsilaterally and rotation of the cervical column contralaterally. Therefore this action of the transversospinalis on the cervical column is analogous to that of the sternomastoid on the head. Thus it is synergistic with the sternomastoid (S.C.O.M.) but, whereas it acts segmentally all along the cervical column, the latter acts on the cervical column as a whole. As its fibres are attached to the two ends of the cervical column it acts upon the column by means of the two arms of a lever.

The **superficial plane** of the posterior neck muscles (fig. 86) consists of the *trapezius* (Tr), which arises fanwise from a line joining the medial third of the superior nuchal line of the occiput, the posterior cervical ligament and the spines of the cervical and thoracic vertebrae down to T_{10}. From their origin the uppermost fibres run an oblique course inferiorly, laterally and anteriorly to be inserted into the lateral third of the clavicle, the acromion and the spine of the scapula. Thus the *contour of the lower part of the neck* is formed by the successive fibres of the trapezius as they curve laterally in oblique fashion. The trapezius is important in moving the scapula (see vol. I) but, when its scapular insertion is stabilised, it acts powerfully on the cervical column and the head, as follows:

when both trapezius muscles contract symmetrically, the cervical column is extended and the cervical lordosis is accentuated. When this extension is counterbalanced by the antagonistic action of the anterior muscles of the neck, they act as *tighteners* that stabilise the whole cervical column;

when only one trapezius contracts (fig. 87: seen from the back; only the left trapezius is shown), *the head is extended and the cervical lordosis is accentuated while it is flexed ipsilaterally and rotated contralaterally.* Thus the trapezius is a synergist of the ipsilateral sterno-mastoid.

In the superior medial corner of the posterior aspect of the neck (fig. 86) the upper extremity of the sterno-mastoid can be seen. Thus the *contour of the upper part of the postero-lateral aspect of the neck is formed by the* successive fibres of the sterno-mastoid as they course inferiorly in different directions and twist about its axis.

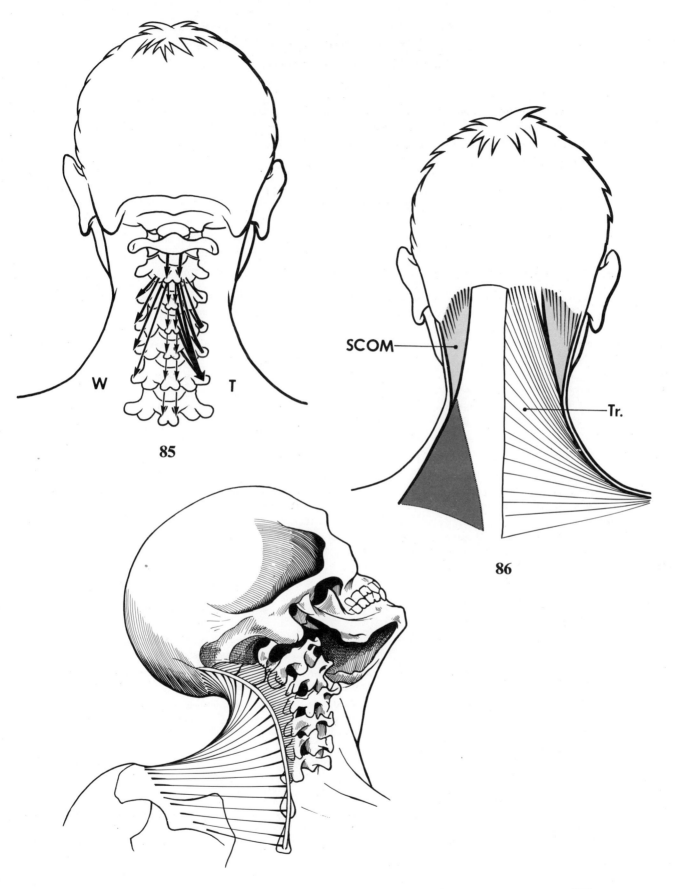

85

86

SCOM

Tr.

87

THE POSTERIOR MUSCLES OF THE NECK:
THE INTERMEDIATE PLANES

Deep to the trapezius is the **third muscular** plane (fig. 88) comprised of the splenius and the levator scapulae.

The **splenius**, which runs from the skull to the thoracic region, arises from the lower six cervical spines, the posterior cervical ligament, the upper four thoracic spines and the interspinous ligament. Its oblique fibres run superiorly, laterally and anteriorly and wrap themselves round the deeper muscles to be inserted as two distinct bands:

the cephalic band, the *splenius capitis* (9), is inserted into the lateral half of the superior nuchal line of the occiput inferior to the sterno-mastoid and into the mastoid process. It incompletely overlies the two semispinalis muscles, which can be seen through the triangle formed by the medial borders of the two splenius muscles;

the cervical band, the *splenius cervicis* (10), is inserted into the transverse processes of the upper three cervical vertebrae (it is shown on the left in relation to the splenius capitis and on the right on its own to show the twist in its fibres).

When these muscles contract bilaterally and symmetrically they extend the head and accentuate the cervical lordosis.

When only one muscle contracts, i.e., *asymmetrically*, it produces the *triple movement of extension, lateral flexion and rotation ipsilaterally*, i.e., the same movement as is typical of the lower cervical column.

The **levator scapulae** (12), lying *lateral to the splenius cervicis*, shares its origin from the transverse processes of the upper four cervical vertebrae. Its flattened belly *twists in the same direction as the splenius* but soon leaves it to run obliquely inferiorly and slightly laterally to gain insertion into the scapula. When its origin is fixed it *elevates the scapula* (see vol. I). On the other hand, if its insertion is kept fixed it moves the cervical column.

When the levators contract bilaterally and symmetrically they extend the cervical column and accentuate the cervical lordosis. If this extension is prevented by their antagonists, then the levators act as *tighteners* to stabilise the cervical column laterally.

When only one levator contracts, i.e., *asymmetrically*, it produces like the splenius *the triple movement of extension, lateral flexion and rotation ipsilaterally*, i.e., the same movement as is typical of the lower cervical column.

The second muscular plane, lying directly on the deep plane, is made up of the semispinalis capitis, the longissimus capitis, the longissimus thoracis, the semispinalis cervicis and the cervical portion of the ilio-costalis.

The **semispinalis capitis** (7), lying just lateral to the midline, forms a vertical muscular band interrupted by an aponeurotic intersection; hence the name 'digastric of the neck'. It arises inferiorly from the transverse processes of the upper six thoracic vertebrae, from the base of the transverse processes of the lower four cervical vertebrae and from the spines of C_7 and T_1. Its muscle belly, thick and rounded, overlies the longisimus capitis and *fills up the vertebral gutter* and is separated from its contralateral homologue by the ligamentum nuchae. The two splenius muscles are closely applied to its lateral convex surface. It is inserted into the squama of the occiput and the medial half of the area between the two nuchal lines.

When the semispinalis muscles contract bilaterally and symmetrically they extend the head and the cervical column and accentuate the cervical lordosis. When one semispinalis contracts, i.e., *asymmetrically, it produces extension with minimal lateral flexion ipsilaterally.*

The **longissimus capitis** (8), lying lateral to the former, is long and thin and runs obliquely superiorly and slightly laterally. It arises from the four lower cervical and the first thoracic transverse processes and is inserted into the posterior border of the mastoid process. Its fibres *twist on themselves* as its lowest fibres are inserted the most medially and vice versa.

When the *longissimus muscles contract bilaterally and symmetrically* they extend the head; when this extension is counterbalanced by the anterior muscles of the neck, they stabilise the head laterally, acting like inverted tighteners.

When *one longissimus muscle contracts*, i.e., *asymmetrically*, it produces *extension and lateral flexion ipsilaterally*, more marked than that produced by the semispinalis capitis, and also *rotation ipsilaterally*.

The **semispinalis cervicis** (11), which is long and thin, lies lateral to the former and arises inferiorly from the transverse processes of T_1–T_5 and is inserted into the transverse processes of C_3–C_7. The deepest fibres, those running between C_7 and T_1, are the shortest, and the most superficial fibres, those running between C_3 and T_5, are the longest.

When *these muscles contract bilaterally and symmetrically they extend the lower cervical column*. If this extension is counterbalanced by their antagonists these muscles act as tighteners.

When *one muscle contracts*, i.e., *asymmetrically, it produces extension and lateral flexion ipsilaterally*.

The **longissimus thoracis** also belongs to the posterior neck muscles by virtue of its uppermost fibres attached to the transverse processes of the lowest cervical vertebrae. It is more or less continuous with the **cervical portion of the ilio-costalis** (11'), which arises from the superior margin of the first six ribs and is inserted, along with the longissimus thoracic, into the posterior tubercle of C_3–C_7. Its actions are similar to those of the longissimus thoracis but in addition it acts as a muscular tightener of the lower cervical column and can elevate the first six ribs (see page 148).

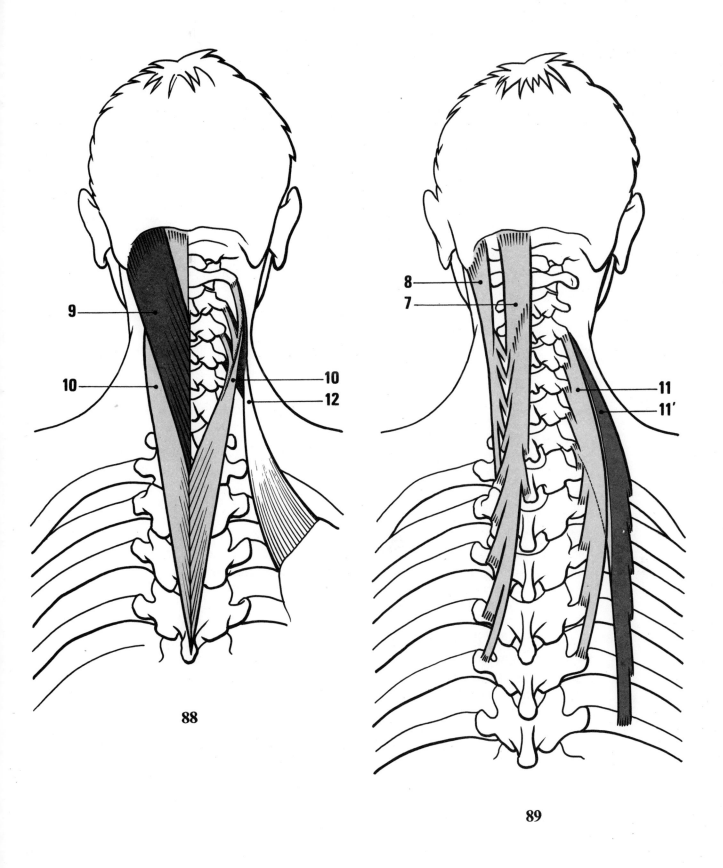

88

89

EXTENSION OF THE CERVICAL COLUMN BY THE POSTERIOR NECK MUSCLES

These muscles all *extend the cervical column and the head* but, depending on their orientation, they can be divided into three groups:

Group I (fig. 90), comprising all the muscles arising from the cervical transverse processes and running obliquely *inferiorly and posteriorly* to the thoracic region:

the *splenius cervicis* (10);

the *semispinalis cervicis* and the cervical portion of the ilio-costalis (11);

the *levator scapulae* (12).

These muscles extend the cervical column and increase the cervical lordosis. When they contract unilaterally they produce extension, *lateral flexion and rotation of the cervical column ipsilaterally*. Thus they produce the composite movement of the lower cervical column (see p. 212).

Group II (fig. 91), comprising all the muscles that run obliquely inferiorly and anteriorly:

on the one hand, the *transverso-spinalis* (5), which is an intrinsic muscle of the lower cervical column;

on the other, the muscles linking the occiput to the lower cervical column: the *semispinalis capitis* (7), the *longissimus capitis* (8) and the *splenius capitis* (not shown in this diagram).

All these muscles *extend the cervical column* and *accentuate the cervical lordosis* and also *extend the head* by virtue of their attachment to the occiput.

Group III comprising all the muscles that *bridge over the cervical column without being attached to its vertebrae*. They connect the occiput and the mastoid process to the scapula. They are:

on the one hand, the *trapezius* (15, fig. 91);

on the other, the sterno-mastoid (fig. 93), which runs diagonally across the cervical column. When the sterno-mastoids contract bilaterally and symmetrically they produce: extension of the head on the cervical column (1), flexion of the cervical on the thoracic column (2) and extension of the cervical column on itself to accentuate the cervical lordosis (3).

The **stability of the cervical column in the sagittal plane** (fig. 93) thus depends on a constant equilibrium between:

on the one hand, extension by the *posterior neck muscles*: splenius (S), ilio-costalis (IC), longissimus thoracis (LT) and trapezius (T); all these muscles spanning completely or partially the cervical curvature;

on the other, the *anterior and antero-lateral muscles—*

the longus capitis (l.c.) which flexes the cervical column and reduces the cervical lordosis;

the scalene muscles (S.c.), which flex the cervical on the thoracic column but which tend to accentuate the cervical lordosis unless they are counteracted by the longus capitis and the supra- and infra-hyoid muscles (see fig. 73).

The simultaneous contraction of all these muscle groups maintains the cervical column rigid in the neutral position. Thus they act like tighteners located in the sagittal plane and in multiple oblique planes. They are therefore essential in *balancing the head* and *in supporting weights carried on the head.*

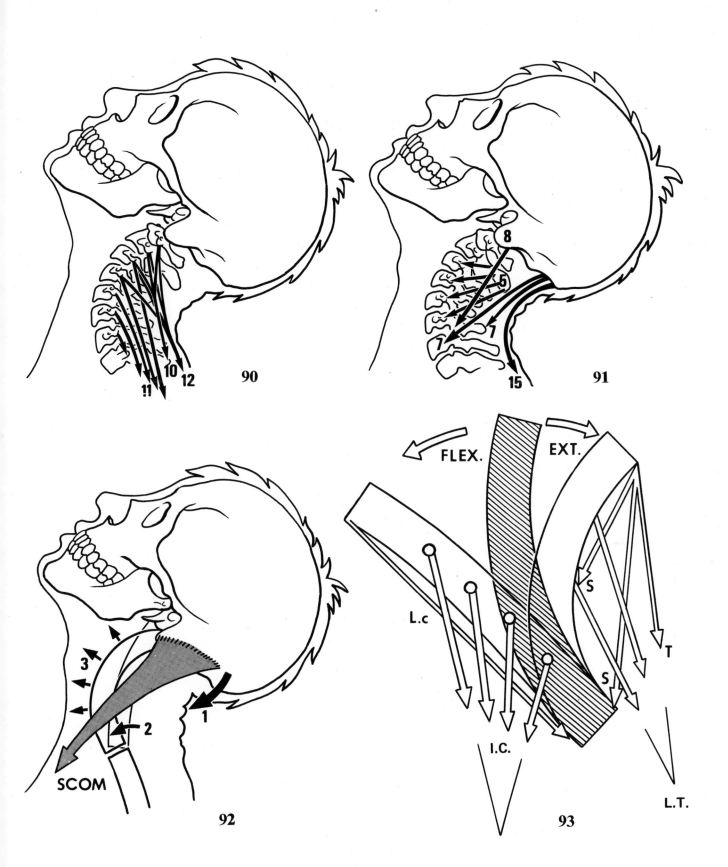

90

91

92

SCOM

93

FLEX.

EXT.

L.c

I.C.

S

S

T

L.T.

243

SYNERGISM AND ANTAGONISM OF PREVERTEBRAL MUSCLES
AND THE STERNO-MASTOID

As already noted (fig. 92), the sterno-mastoids (SCOM) cannot by themselves steady the head and the cervical column. They need the assistance of synergistic and antagonistic muscles that set the stage by first flattening the cervical lordosis (fig. 94). These are:

the *longus capitis* (L.C.) lying just anterior to the vertebral bodies;

the *suboccipital muscles that flex the head on the cervical column* (fig. 95): the rectus capitis anterior and the rectus capitis lateralis;

the *supra- and infra-hyoid muscles*, which lie anterior to the cervical column and act at a distance by means of the long arm of a lever, provided the teeth are clenched by the muscles of mastication.

When the cervical column is held rigid, the cervical lordosis flattened (fig. 96) and extension of the head on the cervical column prevented by the anterior suboccipital muscles and the supra- and infra-hyoid muscles, the two sterno-mastoids (fig. 97) produce *flexion of the cervical column on the thoracic column*. Thus there is synergism-antagonism between the sterno-mastoids and the prevertebral muscles lying against the column or at some distance anteriorly.

244

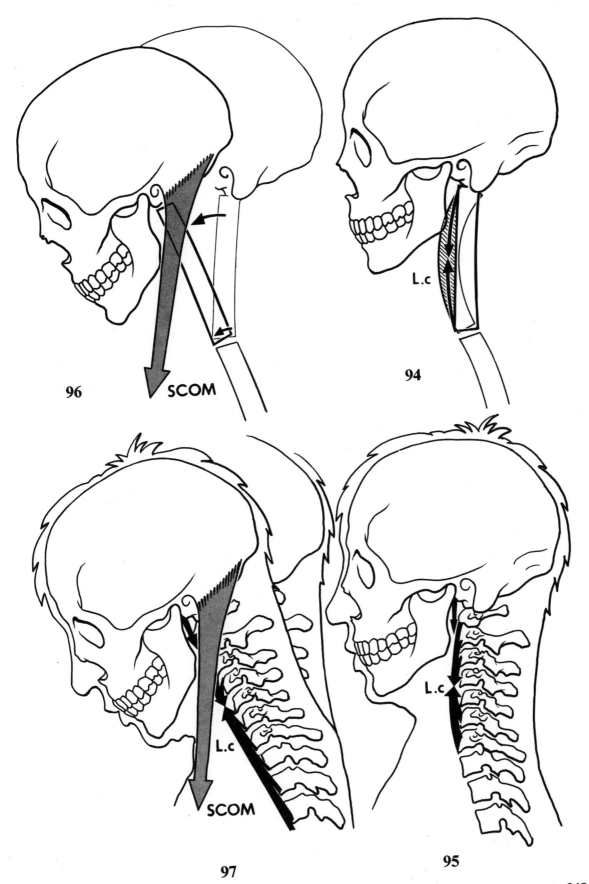

96

SCOM

94

L.c

97

L.c

SCOM

95

L.c

245

THE RANGE OF MOVEMENTS OF THE CERVICAL COLUMN
AS A WHOLE

These ranges can be measured as follows. For flexion and extension and lateral flexion they can be measured accurately on oblique and antero-posterior films but it is more difficult to measure the range of rotation.

Surface markings can also be used and for **flexion and extension** (fig. 98) the *plane of the bite*, which is horizontal in the neutral position, is taken as reference. The angle of extension is that between the plane of the bite and the horizontal and vice versa for flexion. These ranges have already been defined.

For **lateral flexion** (fig. 100) the range is given by the angle formed by *the interclavicular* and *interorbital lines*.

The angle of flexion and extension and lateral flexion can be measured more accurately by placing an *angle-gauge* on the head in the sagittal plane for flexion and extension and in the frontal plane for lateral flexion.

Rotation of the head and neck (fig. 99) can be measured with the subject sitting on a chair and keeping the shoulders steady. The reference plane is then taken as the line of the shoulders and the angle of rotation (R) is measured as the angle formed between the reference plane and the frontal plane passing through the ears, or by the angle (ROT) formed between the sagittal plane of the head and that of the body. More precise measurements can be made with the patient lying flat on his back and an angle-gauge placed on the forehead in the transverse plane.

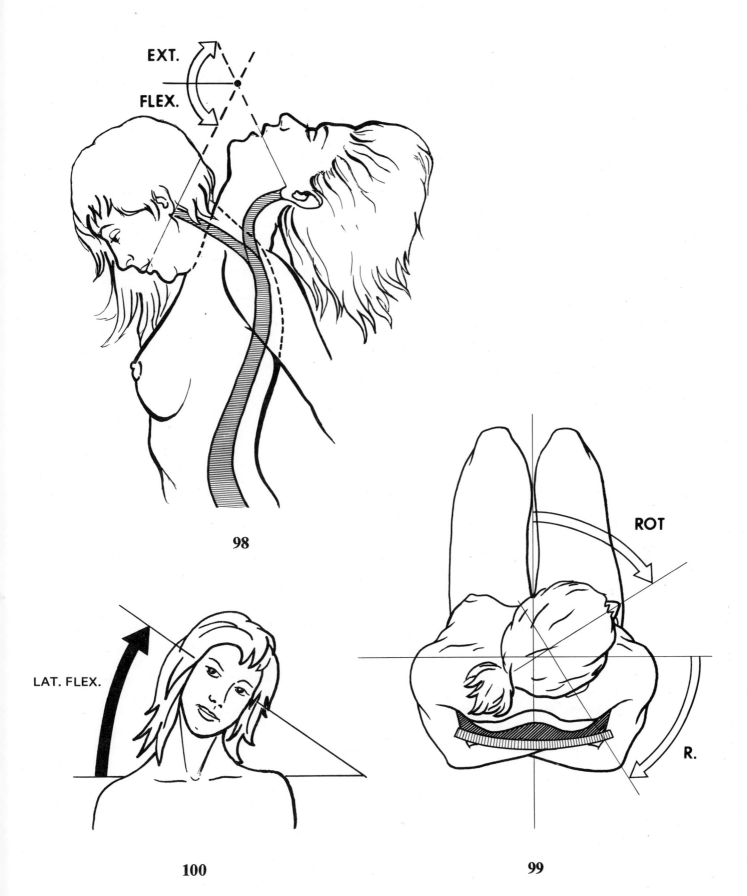

EXT.

FLEX.

98

LAT. FLEX.

100

ROT

R.

99

247

RELATIONSHIP OF THE NEURAXIS TO THE CERVICAL COLUMN

The central nervous system lies within the cranium and the vertebral canal. The cervical column protects the *lower medulla oblongata* as it emerges through the foramen magnum and the *cervical spinal cord* that gives off the nerve roots for the cervical and brachial plexuses. Thus the medulla and the cervical cord are closely related to the highly mobile parts of the cervical column, especially in the suboccipital region which is a highly specialised **zone of mechanical transition** (fig. 101). In fact, as the medualla emerges through the foramen magnum to become the spinal cord (C), it lies *behind and between the two occipital condyldes* which allow the skull to rest on the cervical column. But, between the occipital condyles and C_3, the atlas and the axis will distribute on to three columns the weight of the head, initially supported by two columns (C and C′). These three columns, which extend all along the vertebral column are as follows:

the *main column* (VB) formed by the vertebral bodies and lying anterior to the spinal cord;

the *two lateral columns formed by the articular processes* (A and A′) lying on either side of the cord.

The forces acting on these columns are divided at the level of the *axis which therefore acts as a distributor of forces* between the skull and the atlas, on the one hand, and the rest of the vertebral column, on the other. In fact (fig. 102) the forces acting on each occipital condyle (C) will be divided into two components:

on the one hand, the *main forces operating when the head is at rest* act *on the vertebral bodies* (VB) through the body of the axis;

on the other, the *forces operating during movement* act *on the articular processes* through the pedicle of the axis and its inferior articular facet lying inferior to its posterior arch.

This suboccipital region therefore is at once the pivot, i.e., the most mobile point, of the vertebral column and the area of maximal mechanical activity. This stresses the importance of the ligaments and bones involved in stabilising this region. The most important structure is the *odontoid* and a fracture of the odontoid makes the atlas totally unstable on the axis, which can thus tilt backwards or forwards with the risk of death due to compression of the medulla.

Another important structure for the stability of the atlas on the axis is the *transverse ligament*. If this ligament is torn, the atlas is dislocated anteriorly and the odontoid can press on the medulla causing sudden death. However ruptures of the transverse ligament are less common than fractures of the odontoid.

In the **lower cervical column**, the point of maximal activity is between C_5 and C_6, where anterior dislocations are most frequent with the inferior articular facet of C_5 becoming 'hooked' on to the superior facets of C_6 (fig. 103). In this position the spinal cord is compressed between the vertebral arch of C_6 and the postero-superior border of its vertebral body. Thus depending on the level of cord lesion, paraplegia or quadriplegia, often fatal, may result.

It follows that all these lesions, which render the vertebral column very unstable, can be made worse by *injudicious handling of the injured.* It is particularly important to realise that any flexion of the vertebral column and of the head on the cervical column will aggravate compression of the medulla or cord. Thus, when an injured person is picked up, one of the rescuers must be solely responsible for *keeping the head in the axis of the vertebral column and even to slightly extend it,* so as to prevent the displacement of any broken or dislocated bone at any level of the column.

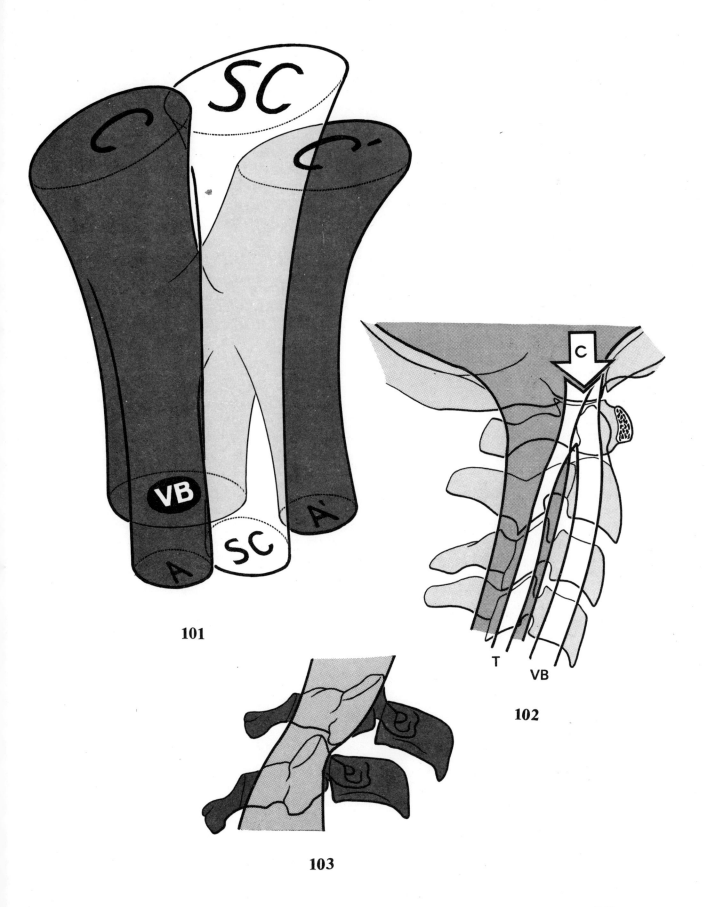

101

102

103

RELATIONSHIP OF THE CERVICAL NERVE ROOTS TO THE CERVICAL COLUMN

At every level of the cervical column nerve *roots emerge from the canal through the intervertebral foramina*. These roots can be involved by *pathological lesions* of the column (fig. 104). Disc prolapse is rare in the cervical region as the discs cannot escape postero-laterally (arrow 1) because of the unciform processes of the vertebral bodies. If disc prolapse occurs (arrow 2), it is more central than in the lumbar region and so tends to cause far more severe cord compression.

Cord compression in the cervical region is more commonly caused by *osteoarthrosis of the unco-vertebral joints* (arrow 3).

Fig. 105 (seen from the side) shows the close relationship between the cervical roots emerging through the intervertebral foramina and the joints between the articular processes posteriorly and the unco-vertebral joints anteriorly. During the development of osteoarthrosis (the bottom part of the figure) osteophytes not only appear on the anterior border of the vertebral plateaus but *they are more frequently seen at the level of the unco-vertebral joints projecting into the confines of the intervertebral foramen*. Also osteophytes grow posteriorly *from the joints between the articular processes* and the nerve roots may be compressed by osteophytes arising anteriorly from the unco-vertebral joints and posteriorly from the joints between the articular processes. This explains the symptomatology of cervical osteoarthrosis.

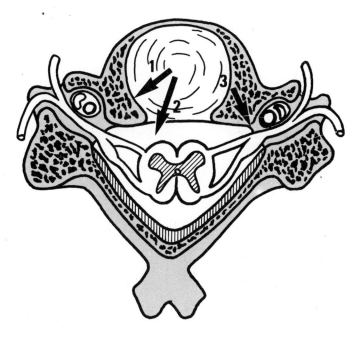

104

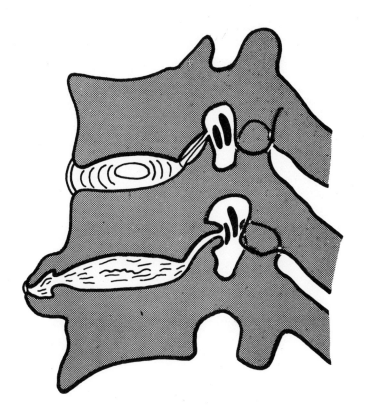

105